Why migraine sufferers are choosing
Overcoming Migraine as their guide

Doctors and therapists respond:

Overcoming Migraine should be required reading for every patient and therapist. Betsy Wyckoff offers a guidebook that couples an impressive compendium of information with a sensitive awareness of the headache sufferer's treatment needs.

Jan Bennett, M.A.
Supervisor, Muscle Tension Therapy
Neurologic Centre for Headache and Pain, La Jolla, California

A simply written book that provides information on migraine that is readily understandable. Recommended for basic facts on this disorder.

Seymour Diamond, M.D.
Director, Diamond Headache Clinic, Chicago, Illinois
Executive Director, National Headache Foundation

Readers respond:

I almost cried as I read the first page because I did not feel so alone anymore. It was as if you were writing about me.

D.L., Lawrenceville, Georgia

It is good to know I am not alone. Thank you for your wonderful and informative book.

Dusty Hardman, Estes Park, Colorado

Your book is the most helpful I have ever read on the subject, and believe me, I've read them all. It is comprehensive yet succinct, though not so clipped as to deny the person behind the headache.

Betty, Ohio

When I first read the book I thought that, even if I didn't get over my headaches, you at least had given me, and, I'm sure, countless other women, the guts to stand up to my doctor, be taken seriously, or find one who would take me seriously . . . . Thank you again for your fine book.

G.N., Seattle, Washington

I was most impressed with your chapter on m____ ___ nd hormones. You are the first person w¹ ___ e seems to be a connection (between) m¹ ___ e."

____ Vorth, Texas

It was a great relief to read ___ :al condition rather than a mental aberrati ___ ___ can find about this condition and appreciate the common-sense approach of your book.

Ruth C. Sillman, Meriden, Connecticut

I find this guide to be an excellent reference, as I easily confuse the mechanisms that trigger headaches and cause them to linger . . . . You may be interested to know that I have sent copies of the book to other friends with migraine problems.

Alice Helpern, New York, New York

I wish that more people were aware of the severity of migraine. I hated being treated as though I were a crybaby who enjoys complaining and using my headaches as an excuse to miss work and gain sympathy. As you know, this was not the case. I found your book helpful since I realized that many others are treated in the same manner, and that we have to be aggressive about our treatment. We do not deserve to live with this pain and frustration, and we should not stand for it. I never will again, and I will urge others with migraines to persist until they have found effective medications, as you did.

Darcie M. Cournoyer, Duxbury, Massachusetts

Your book has been of great help regarding food and other triggers . . . . Thank you for your contribution to the welfare of many.

A.C.M., Santo Domingo, Dominican Republic

I learned a good deal from your book and could see bits and pieces of myself in your personal migraine history . . . . I appreciate *Overcoming Migraine* and the contribution I am sure it will make in finding a cure for migraines.

Virginia Leigh Hiles, Pass Christian, Missouri

Thank you for tackling this enormous controversy and trying to make some sense out of it.

Jo Anne Marquardt, Sacramento, California

I received so much help from your fine work.

Sister M.C., Ft. Smith, Arizona

You have made the lives of those suffering from migraine attacks more tolerable. Hopefully, you have stimulated additional research by your excellent compendium.

H.W.C., Ph.D., Davis, California

You may have saved my sanity.

Mindie Dolson, Oakdale, California

I am amazed at the wealth of information and research you have put in this book . . . . You have covered everything. The book will help so many migraine sufferers — we all thank you.

L.O., New York, New York

REVISED & EXPANDED EDITION

Overcoming Migraine

A Comprehensive Guide to Treatment and Prevention by a Survivor

Betsy Wyckoff

P·U·L·S·E
Station Hill Press

A P.U.L.S.E. Book, published by Station Hill Press, Inc., Barrytown, New York 12507.

Text and cover design by Susan Quasha, assisted by Vicki Hickman.

Distributed in the United States and Canada by the Talman Company, 131 Spring Street, Suite 201E-N, New York, New York 10012.

Library of Congress Cataloging-in-Publication Data

Wyckoff, Betsy.
 Overcoming Migraine: a compreshensive guide to treatment and prevention by a survivor / Betsy Wyckoff.
  p. cm.
 "Revised & expanded."
 Includes bibliographical references and index.
 ISBN 0-88268-163-X : $10.95
 1. Migraine–Popular works. I. Title.
RC392.W93   1993
616.8 ' .57–dc20
                                                            93-35705
                                                            CIP

Manufactured in the United States of America.

Acknowledgments

I would like to thank the National Headache Foundation in Chicago, the Migraine Foundation of Canada in Toronto, the Migraine Trust in London, and the Australian Bureau of Statistics for the migraine population figures in the Introduction. I would also like to thank the Migraine Trust for their help in the preparation of the list of headache clinics in the United Kingdom and Australia in Appendix III.

I would like to thank the National Headache Foundation and Wyeth-Ayerst Laboratories for permission to use the art from the "Migraine Masterpieces" exhibition. All of the art in this book was created by artists who are migraine sufferers.

Note to the Reader

Although the author has researched all sources thoroughly to ensure the accuracy of the information contained in this book, she assumes no responsibility for inaccuracies or omissions contained herein. Symptoms of, and tests for, the disorders discussed as well as drug dosages, side effects, precautions, interactions, and contra-indications should be confirmed by the reader in consultation with his or her personal physician.

Contents

This book is dedicated to my mother, Pauline, who suffered in silence, and to Julie for her support of my effort to combat this disorder.

Introduction

Approximately 18 million people in the United States, over 4 million people in Canada, 5 million people in the United Kingdom, and almost 231 thousand people in Australia suffer from migraine headaches. I am one of these people. I had intermittent migraines for twenty-five years before my daily migraines began. I experienced nausea and vomiting every day for three months and was finally diagnosed as having atypical migraine. This period was followed by five months of daily migraine headaches.

Life seemed hardly worth living. Eventually I became angry—angry at the pain, my doctors, and the side effects of the drugs I was taking. Mostly, I was angry at my own ignorance. I determined to research every bit of information existing on this condition. I read medical textbooks and journal articles as well as the more holistic fringe literature. All of the information I found is presented in this book. Because I believe people in pain do not have the patience to wade through a lengthy tome, I have organized my research findings as well as my own story into a concise presentation.

This book is the answer to the many questions I had about my migraines. I believe these are questions you, too, must have asked about your headaches.

First and foremost, I wondered if any migraine medications existed whose side effects were not worse than the headache itself. I describe my search for these drugs in chapters 1 and 2. This material points out how horrendous the hunt for migraine medications can be if neither you nor your doctor knows very much about migraine treatment. The main purpose of these chapters is to help you become familiar with the various classes of migraine medications.

Next, I wondered if changes in my diet, environment, or lifestyle would help my headaches. Migraine triggers are discussed in chapters 3 and 4.

I thought my headaches might be a symptom of some other disease. The results of my search for disorders that can be accompanied by headache are outlined in chapter 5.

Since my headaches were worse during menstruation and menopause, I researched the connection between hormones and migraine. My findings are summarized in chapter 6.

At times I thought I had muscle contraction headaches and not migraines at all. I discuss the difference between these two kinds of headaches in chapter 7.

Biofeedback and other nonpharmacological treatments are explored in chapter 8.

Who are the experts in migraine management and how do you go about finding them? My answers to these questions are in chapter 9. The results of my inquiries into migraine prevention and treatment are summarized in chapter 10.

Additional questions have come to mind since the first edition of this book went to press. These questions are explored in the second edition of the book. The first edition concerned migraine in the adult, but what about migraine in children and the elderly? How migraine and its treatment differs in these age groups is discussed in chapters 11 and 12, respectively. I also wondered if any anecdotal or unorthodox treatments existed that were not covered in the traditional migraine literature. These treatments are reviewed in chapters 13 and 14. A request for information from the reader was published in the first edition of the book. Replies to this request can be found in chapter 15.

The dose, precautions, and side effects of various migraine medications are outlined in Appendix I. The physiology of migraine is discussed throughout the book. I pull all of this information into one place in Appendix II. Headache clinics in the United States, Canada, the United Kingdom, and Australia are listed in Appendix III. A list of migraine associations can be found in Appendix IV.

I feel I have touched upon everything that is known about migraine prevention and treatment. It is my firm belief that this book contains all the information needed to help you overcome this dreadful disorder. Be persistent. Have hope. A life free of pain is possible if you are willing to take action.

1

A Personal Migraine History

I first experienced migraine symptoms in my early twenties. I would get from two to three headaches every month, with one of these headaches coinciding with menstruation. Each headache would increase in severity throughout the day and would last approximately fourteen hours. The pain was located above my right eye and was throbbing in nature. My right nostril was stuffy and would run when the headache broke. At times the headache seemed to imitate a sinus infection. I had no nausea or vomiting, as is sometimes the case. I came to learn that what I had was labeled a "common" migraine, as opposed to the "classic" migraine in which there are visual symptoms, such as flashing lights, preceding the headache.

During one excruciating bout I went to my local hospital's emergency room where I was given Tylenol with codeine for the pain. The emergency room physician made appointments for me to have an electroencephalogram (EEG) and to see a neurologist. The EEG was negative. The neurologist told me my headache was caused by "nerves." I was so angry at being dismissed as just another neurotic female that I decided I would investigate headaches on my own. Fortunately, my local bookstore has a medical department with a well-stocked neurology section. In one of the textbooks I bought, I found a sentence stating that migraines could be caused by foods containing tyramine, a vasodilator. I was able to get a list of these foods, and when I stayed away from them, I had headaches only during menstruation.[1]

My headaches remained minimal until I reached menopause. During the first year of menopause I was free of headaches and I ate foods containing tyramine with fierce abandon. In January of my third year after starting menopause, I began a period of daily nausea and vomiting that lasted for three months.

My internist sent me for a series of tests, thinking a gall bladder ailment was the cause of my symptoms. The upper GI series and abdominal ultrasound revealed no disease. Since a brain tumor can cause nausea and vomiting, I had a brain scan using magnetic resonance imaging (MRI), which also revealed no tumor or other malady.

In the meantime, I had been taking a variety of antiemetic drugs. Of these, Compazine, Dramamine, Tigan, and Emetrol had little effect. Phenergan did seem to help the nausea to some extent, but I was unable to eat because of the nausea and lost almost 30 pounds in three months.

My internist referred me to a gastroenterologist who performed an endoscopic exam. This test was also negative. Because migraine runs in my family, the gastroenterologist diagnosed my symptoms as atypical migraine in which the nausea and vomiting masked an underlying migraine headache. He also felt I had status migrainosus in which one headache triggered the next, causing the symptoms to continue from day to day. I was given Torecan by this doctor. This antiemetic drug controlled the nausea more than any other medication I had tried.

Because my problem was now diagnosed as migraine, I returned to my internist to begin a series of treatments with traditional migraine medications. These treatments will be discussed in chapter 2.

In summary, over a period of twenty-five years, the frequency of my migraine headaches increased from approximately one a month to a three-month period of atypical migraine consisting of daily nausea and vomiting. Diagnosis was difficult and time-consuming because at this point I had no headache, only nausea.

---

1. These foods will be discussed in chapter 3.

2

Beginning Treatment

Such analgesics as aspirin, acetaminophen (Tylenol), and ibuprofen (Advil, Nuprin, Mediprin) did little to alleviate my symptoms. Like aspirin and ibuprofen, Anaprox (naproxen) is an anti-inflammatory drug with analgesic properties. Many migraine sufferers find it to be an effective pain medication. Paradoxically, Anaprox intensified my symptoms.

The pain of migraine comes from vascular dilation. Ergotamine is used to treat migraine because of its vasoconstricting properties. The drug comes from a fungus that grows on rye. Ergotamine can be obtained in oral and sublingual tablets, in suppository form, as an aerosol, or can be administered by injection. Ergotamine should be taken at the very beginning of a migraine attack.

The side effects of ergotamine include nausea and, in cases where use is excessive, gangrene of the limbs. If taken for two days in a row, ergotamine may produce a rebound headache. Because the headache underlying my symptoms of nausea and vomiting was continual, my doctor prescribed Bellergal-S which contains such a small amount of ergotamine it can be taken every day. Bellergal-S also contains phenobarbital, which is a sedative, as well as an ingredient to counteract the nausea caused by the ergotamine. The phenobarbital caused a paradoxical reaction in that it made me hyperactive. Bellergal-S, probably because of its low dose of ergotamine, did little to reverse my symptoms. However, for many people who only get migraines two or three times a month, ergotamine can be taken in a high enough dose to be an effective abortive agent.

The process that causes a headache is thought to begin with a period of vasoconstriction that is triggered by the release of serotonin, a neurotransmitter. As serotonin is absorbed, the amount is depleted. Lower serotonin levels produce vasodilation and headache. Since this process is triggered by the release of serotonin, any drug that regulates serotonin would be of value in migraine prevention. An antidepressant is just such a drug.

My doctor prescribed two antidepressants for me. Elavil (amitriptyline), the first, made me feel as if the skin were coming off my bones. The second antidepressant, Tofranil (imipramine), made me very jittery. Antidepressants were ruled out, and we next tried Fiorinal.

Fiorinal contains a barbiturate, aspirin, and caffeine. The sedative and muscle relaxant effects of Fiorinal are helpful in the treatment of tension headaches. Fiorinal did little to alleviate my migraine symptoms.

I was becoming desperate. My nausea was continuing, and no treatment was helping the migraine underlying the nausea. At this point I asked my internist to recommend a neurologist.

The first thing the neurologist did was to prescribe Reglan (metoclopramide) for my nausea. Nausea is often associated with a delay of gastric emptying, and thus prevents many migraine medications from being properly absorbed. Reglan relieves nausea and enhances the absorption of migraine medications because it increases gastric emptying. It has become the drug of choice in treating the nausea that may accompany migraine. Reglan can cause trembling as well as anxiety, but these side effects are usually transitory.

The neurologist's next major effort was to treat my atypical migraine, which had developed into a daily experience known as status migrainosus. By now I had had constant nausea and vomiting, but no headaches, for almost three months. The doctor prescribed prednisone, a steroid, for five days. Nothing happened. We waited for one week and tried the prednisone a second time. Again nothing happened. On the third course of prednisone my nausea disappeared and I began to experience the migraine that had been masked by the nausea. Daily migraine attacks were not aborted by additional prednisone.

In the meantime, I was treating the migraine with Tylenol and codeine. Although codeine is a narcotic, addiction to the drug is rare if it is not used on a daily basis. I was afraid of this drug and only used it when my symptoms became intolerable. I had previously used Tylenol and codeine for the nausea after the doctor convinced me that, even though I felt no pain, I should treat the nausea as a headache. He was right. The medication alleviated the nausea.

The beta blocking agents are used to treat heart problems as well as hypertension. Studies of patients with migraines revealed that some of these agents also prevent migraine attacks. Inderal (propranolol), Corgard (nadolol), Blocadren (timolol), Tenormin (atenolol), and Lopressor (metoprolol) are used in the treatment of migraine, with Inderal being the most effective of these agents. It is not known how beta-blockers work to prevent migraine, but it is thought that one of their characteristics is to prevent the dilation of blood vessels.

The gastroenterologist, once he suspected migraine as the cause of my nausea, had prescribed Inderal for me. The drug stopped my symptoms, which confirmed his diagnosis of migraine. However, I could not tolerate the drug's side effects of breathlessness, fatigue, lethargy, and insomnia. The neurologist I was now seeing wanted me to try Corgard since we knew that at least one of the beta blocking class of drugs had worked for me. This drug penetrates the central nervous system poorly so it rarely causes insomnia. A trial run of Corgard proved to be ineffective in my case.

In spite of my experience, Inderal and the other beta blockers have proven to be some of the most powerful prophylatic agents used in migraine treatment. Inderal can be obtained in a sustained-released capsule that is administered once daily. It should be noted that patients with certain heart conditions, asthma, or diabetes cannot be treated with some of the beta blockers. Asthmatics and diabetics seem to react less strongly to Tenormin and Lopressor.

Sansert (methysergide) is another migraine medication that prevents headaches by inhibiting serotonin and constricting blood vessels. One of the many side effects of the drug is fibrosis or the forming of scar-like tissue in the heart and lungs. Sansert should be discontinued one month out of four to prevent this complication.

Although I have never taken LSD, Sansert (which is related to LSD) made me feel as if I was on a bad trip, with hallucinations being my major complaint. I was so frightened by my reaction to the drug that I went to a local hospital's emergency room for help. Before the emergency room staff got around to me, four hours had elapsed, and the effects of the drug had started to wear off. I left in disgust and swore to investigate the migraine medications I was taking with more diligence. As it turns out, I am one of the people that cannot tolerate Sansert. Although often a drug of last resort, Sansert has helped some migraine sufferers.

The calcium channel blockers dilate blood vessels. By blocking cellular calcium, they prevent the original constriction of the vessels by stopping the calcium needed for this reaction. As mentioned earlier, it is vasodilation in reaction to vasoconstriction that causes the head to ache.

My neurologist prescribed the calcium channel blocker Isoptin (verapamil) for me. I thought I was going to have a stroke on this drug. My head felt as if it were going to explode. The pressure was so intense I refused to continue using the drug. I could literally "feel" the vasodilating properties of Isoptin. I later learned that the calcium channel blockers are best taken when the cerebral arteries are in a state of rest, not after the headache has begun.

In spite of my experiences, these fairly new medications are considered by some headache specialists to hold much promise in the treatment of migraine. Other migraine specialists feel that the calcium channel blockers have been overrated in the prophylaxis of migraine because of their side effects and the long period needed before their effect is felt.

The doctor was beginning to understand that I react with great sensitivity to many migraine medications. Perhaps as a result, he next prescribed feverfew, a drug made from the dried leaves of a plant in the daisy family, *Tanacetum parthenium*. Feverfew can be obtained in most health food stores. It has anti-inflammatory properties and is thought to inhibit serotonin. In a very small percentage of users, feverfew's side effects include mouth ulcers, itchy skin, and a sore throat.

The leaves of the feverfew plant are freeze-dried and appear in capsule form. The usual dose is 125 mg once daily.[1] It is suggested that the herb not be used if you drink alcohol or are taking high blood pressure medicine. Painkillers retard the herb's effect, which may be why it did little to alter my headaches.

---

1. Hancock, K. (1986): *Feverfew: Your Headache May Be Over.* New Canaan, Connecticut : Keats Publishing.

Feverfew first became popular in England, and hundreds of migraine sufferers in that country testify to its value. It is especially appreciated because, unlike so many drugs used in migraine prevention, the side effects are minimal.

The neurologist told me his next plan was to give me anticonvulsive medication. Anticonvulsant drugs, such as Tegretol (carbamazepine) and Dilantin (phenytoin), have been used for many years to treat children with migraine, but the use of these drugs to treat adult migraine patients is controversial. Published studies using anticonvulsant drugs to treat migraine in nonepileptic adults are meager, although anecdotal reports do exist. Due to my previous experience with medications, the side effects of these drugs made me very wary. I felt my doctor was grasping at straws. Before taking any more drugs, I decided it was time for me to get another opinion. By now my headaches had continued on a daily basis, in one form or another, for over eight months.

I first went to the headache clinic at the Montefiore Medical Center in Bronx, New York. After an extensive examination, the neurologist suggested I try Inderal, Anaprox, and Midrin. He felt I should use Inderal as an abortive agent in which I would take only the morning dose, and in this way I might avoid the side effects that accompanied Inderal in the past. Inderal taken in this fashion has, at times, bought me up to eight hours of headache relief.

Anaprox used on a daily basis has been found to prevent headaches. However, I was one of the 5 percent of the people in whom the drug produced headaches.

Midrin contains isometheptene mucate (a vasoconstrictor), dichloralphenazone (a mild sedative), and acetaminophen (an analgesic). It is a good abortive agent for mild to moderate migraine. Midrin is similar to ergotamine in its actions but has less severe side effects. For example, Midrin does not cause nausea. It also does not produce rebound headaches. The usual dose is 2 capsules to start.[1] These may be followed by 1 capsule every hour up to 5 per day.[2] Do not exceed 15 capsules per week.[3] I found Midrin to be one of the more successful drugs that had been prescribed for my migraines.

---

1. Diamond, S. and Millstein, E. (1988): Current concepts of migraine therapy. *Journal of Clinical Pharmacology* 28: 195.

2. Ibid.

3. Ibid.

My next step was to call the National Headache Foundation in Chicago to request their physician membership list for my area. The number in Illinois is 1-800-523-8858; outside of Illinois the number is 1-800-843-2256. I felt that any neurologist who belonged to the foundation would be particularly interested in headaches.

The next neurologist that I saw prescribed lithium for me. Lithium is used for chronic cluster headaches. Its use for migraine is controversial. People on lithium must be closely supervised. A high blood level can cause shakiness or confusion. Long time use can cause kidney and thyroid problems. In some cases, lithium makes migraine worse. On the other hand, lithium seems to help people with cyclic migraine in whom headaches occur daily for six weeks or so and then stop for several weeks. Because this was not the pattern of my headaches, I decided to put lithium on hold for a while.

After reviewing all of the drugs used in migraine treatment, I realized I had not explored the tricyclic antidepressants thoroughly. I knew that although I could not tolerate Elavil or Tofranil, that did not mean I would have the same experience with other drugs in this class. Aventyl (nortriptyline) and Sinequan (doxepin) are two of several antidepressants reported to prevent migraine headaches. Sinequan and Tofranil inhibit both serotonin and norepinephrine, Aventyl mainly inhibits norepinephrine, and Elavil acts primarily as an inhibitor of serotonin.

Sinequan has turned out to be a good migraine prophylactic medication for me. Because it can cause drowsiness, Sinequan is taken once a day at bedtime. I have a reverse reaction in that instead of drowsiness, as little as 10 mg can cause increased energy levels and insomnia. For this reason, I take Sinequan in the morning. I now believe if I had taken only 10 mg of Elavil, instead of 25 mg, I might have found headache relief months earlier.

Catapres (clonidine) is one drug used in the treatment of migraine that I have not tried. It is normally used to treat high blood pressure. Catapres should be discontinued slowly to prevent hypertension. The side effects of this drug include dry mouth, drowsiness, and dizziness. It has been found to be disappointing in migraine treatment. In some studies it was no more effective than a placebo.

Periactin (cyproheptadine) blocks histamine and serotonin receptors. It is primarily used to treat migraine in children but has been helpful in some cases of adult migraine. I have not used this drug because I have a paradoxical reaction to antihistamines in that they cause headaches rather than prevent them. Periactin cannot be combined with alcohol or MAO inhibitors. It can cause seizures in epileptics. Its side effects in adults include sedation, weight gain, dizziness, and dry mouth.

Dihydroergotamine (DHE) nasal spray and pizotifen are two migraine medications not available in the United States. DHE nasal spray has shown promise in aborting the occasional migraine. DHE nasal spray is rapidly absorbed and has fewer side effects than other ergotamine preparations. Pizotifen is a preventative migraine medication. Although the drug helps some people, not all migraine sufferers who take pizotifen find it effective. The drug's side effects include increased appetite and drowsiness.

Sumatriptan, a new drug which has been effective in treating migraine during clinical trials, is a vasconstrictor similiar to ergotamine. Unlike ergotamine, it does not cause nausea and its effectiveness is not dependent on taking the drug at the beginning of a migraine attack. Clinical trials in Europe showed that 70 percent of the people taking sumatriptan orally and 85 percent of those taking it by subcutaneous injection aborted their migraine attacks within 30 to 60 minutes. Sumatriptan is available in Britain and the Netherlands under the brand name Imigran. The injectable form of sumatriptan (Imitrex) has been approved for use in the United States.

Each migraine sufferer reacts to the drugs discussed in this chapter differently. In my case I have found Midrin to be helpful in aborting a migraine once it has begun. If the headache is not completely aborted, I take Tylenol with codeine in addition to Midrin. Abortive medications are listed in Table 2.1.

Table 2.1
Abortive Medications

MEDICATION	INGREDIENTS	COMMENTS
Analgesics		
Aspirin	Acetylsalicylic acid 227-400 mg. (May be combined with acetaminophen, caffeine, or buffers)	Overuse many cause internal bleeding. Buffers reduce stomach irritation

MEDICATION	INGREDIENTS	COMMENTS
Advil, Nuprin, Medipren	Ibuprofen 200 mg	More than 1000 mg per day of aspirin or Tylenol can cause rebound headaches
Tylenol	Acetaminophen 325 or 500 mg	
Tylenol with codeine	Acetaminophen 300 mg, codeine phosphate 7.5, 15, 30 and 60 mg	Can cause habituation

Nonsteroidal anti-inflammatory

Anaprox	Naproxen sodium 275 mg	Take with food or antacid to prevent nausea

Ergotamine

Cafergot (oral)	Ergotamine tartrate 1 mg, caffeine 100 mg	Continual use can cause rebound headaches. Do not exceed 6 tablets per day or 10 tablets per week of oral dose.[1] Do not exceed 2 suppositories per day or 5 suppositories per week of rectal dose [2]
Cafergot (rectal)	Ergotamine tartrate 2 mg, caffeine 100 mg	
Wigraine (oral)	Ergotamine tartrate 1 mg, caffeine 100 mg	
Wigraine (rectal)	Ergotamine tartrate 2 mg, caffeine 100 mg	
Medihaler Ergotamine (aerosol)	Ergotamine tartrate. One dose contains 0.36 mg	The aerosol is no longer on the market in the United States. It is available in Canada, Europe, and the United Kingdom

---

1. Diamond, S. and Millstein, E. (1988): Current concepts of migraine therapy. *Journal of Clinical Pharmacology* 28: 195.
2. Ibid.

MEDICATION	INGREDIENTS	COMMENTS
Ergomar, Ergostat (sublingual)	Ergotamine tartrate 2 mg	One tablet at onset to be repeated every 30 minutes.[1] Do not exceed 3 per day or 5 per week[2]
Midrin	Isometheptene mucate 65 mg, dichloralphenazone 100mg, acetaminophen 325 mg	Take 2 capsules at onset followed by 1 capsule every hour up to 5.[3] Do not exceed 5 capsules per day or 15 per week[4]
Beta Blocker		
Inderal	Propranolol 10, 20, 40, 60, or 80 mg	As little as 10 mg may abort headache
Antiemetic		
Reglan	Metoclopramide 10 mg	
Sumatriptan		
Imitrex (USA) Imigran (UK, the Netherlands)		Check with your doctor about status of availability of sumatriptan in tablet or injectable form

Prophylactic drugs are appropriate for people who get more than one or two migraines each week. These medications are taken daily to prevent a headache from even beginning. I have found the antidepressant drug Sinequan to be effective in eliminating my migraine headaches. The more common prophylactic drugs used in the treatment of migraine are listed in Table 2.2.

1. Ibid.
2. Ibid.
3. Ibid.
4. Ibid.

In summary, throughout the course of three months of nausea and five months of daily migraine, I became a test subject for various migraine medications. To be well informed before starting treatment study the drugs listed in Table 2.1 and Table 2.2.

The drugs listed in Table 2.1 will stop a migraine attack once it has started. There are six major drug groups in this category: analgesics, anti-inflammatories, ergotamine compounds, Midrin, the beta blockers, and sumatriptan. The prophylactic drugs listed in Table 2.2 are taken daily to prevent headaches from arising. They are appropriate if you get migraines on a weekly basis. The five most effective groups of drugs in this category are: the beta blockers, anti-inflammatory drugs, antidepressants, Sansert and the calcium channel blockers.

Table 2.2

Prophylactic Medications

MEDICATION	INGREDIENTS	COMMENTS
Beta blockers		
Inderal	Propranolol hydrochloride 10, 20, 40, 60, 80 mg	Inderal is the most effective of the beta blockers
Corgard	Nadolol 40, 80, 120, 160 mg	Insulin-using diabetics and asthmatics do better on Tenormin or Lopressor
Lopressor	Metoprolol tartrate 50, 100 mg	
Blocadren	Timolol maleate 10, 20 mg	
Tenormin	Atenolol 50, 100 mg	Corgard and Tenormin produce less insomnia

MEDICATION	INGREDIENTS	COMMENTS

Ergotamine

Bellergal	Ergotamine tartrate 0.3 mg, phenobarbital 20 mg, belladonna 0.1 mg	
Bellergal-S	Ergotamine tartrate 0.6 mg, phenobarbital 40 mg, belladonna 0.2 mg	

Nonsteroidal anti-inflammatories

Anaprox	Naproxen sodium 275 mg	Take with food or antacid to prevent nausea
Naprosyn	Naproxen 250, 375, 500 mg	

Antidepressants

Elavil	Amitriptyline hydrochloride 10, 25, 50, 75, 100, 150 mg	
Aventyl	Nortriptyline hydrochloride 10, 25, 50, 75 mg	
Sinequan	Doxepin hydrochloride 10, 25, 50, 75, 100, 150 mg	
Nardil	Phenelzine sulfate 15 mg	MAO inhibitor. Avoid foods containing tyramine

MEDICATION	INGREDIENTS	COMMENTS
Sansert	Methysergide maleate 2 mg	Must be stopped after 4 months to prevent fibrosis. Side effects are common
Calcium channel blockers		
Isoptin	Verapamil hydrochloride 80, 120 mg	Vasodilators
Procardia	Nifedipine 10 mg	
Periactin	Cyproheptadine hydrochloride 4 mg	Antihistamine. Used in treating childhood migraine
Feverfew	*Tanacetum parthenium* 125 mg	Do not take with high dosage high blood pressure medicine or alcohol. Herb. Obtain in health food stores. Dosage is 125 mg per day [1]

---

1. Hancock, K. (1986): *Feverfew: Your Headache May Be Over*. New Canaan, Connecticut: Keats Publishing.

3

Diet and Migraine

People subject to migraines often do not metabolize amines properly. They seem to lack the enzyme necessary to break down these substances. Amines influence the diameter of the blood vessels. Dilated blood vessels produce the pain we know as headache. Tyramine (cheese), phenylethylamine (chocolate), and octopamine (citrus) are examples of the amines in our diet that may trigger a headache.

Nitrites are used as a food preservative. They also trigger headaches in some people, and foods containing this chemical should be avoided. Nitrites may be found in hot dogs, bacon, ham, salami, bologna, sausage, pepperoni, and many other packaged meats.

Foods containing the sugar substitute aspartame are known to produce headaches. Saccharin, on the other hand, is not a migraine trigger. Monosodium glutamate (MSG) is used to enhance the flavor of instant rice, soups, and Chinese food. MSG will precipitate a headache in many people.

Although not listed in the literature as a migraine precipitant, I have found the preservative sodium benzoate to be a migraine trigger.

Reading food labels is extremely important. For example, I was surprised when I got a migraine after eating a cream cheese-smoked salmon dip, since cream cheese is one of the few cheeses that does not contain tyramine. I then read the label on the package only to discover that this product contains MSG. The morning after eating a dinner of steak, rice, and salad, I awoke with a pounding migraine. I read the label on the steak sauce and salad dressing that I had had the night before to discover that both contained the preservative sodium benzoate, a powerful migraine trigger in my case. I could have avoided this headache if I had been in the habit of reading food labels.

Foods containing amines, nitrites, aspartame, MSG, or sodium benzoate should be avoided by many people prone to headaches. These foods are listed in Table 3.1.

Table 3.1

Foods Containing Amines and Other Substances Known to Trigger Headaches

Fruits

Citrus	Avocados
Bananas	Papaya
Canned figs	Pineapples
Dates	Red plums
Raisins	Raspberries
Strawberries	Mangoes

Vegetables

Spinach	Italian broad beans
Lima beans	Pea pods
Soybeans	Sauerkraut
Onions	Fava beans
Garbanzo beans	Lentils
Olives	Snow peas
Pinto beans	Pickles
Navy beans	Tomato
Eggplant	

Meats

Turkey	Game meats
Liver, sweetbreads, kidneys, brains	Salted or smoked fish (lox, anchovies)

Pickled herring

Pork

Preserved meat

Caviar

Chicken livers, pâté

Milk products

Cream

Yogurt

Cheese (except cream cheese and cottage cheese)

Sour cream

Buttermilk

Chocolate

Alcohol

Beer

Sherry

Red wine

Yeast

Fresh coffee cake

Homemade breads

Brewer's yeast

Doughnuts

Sourdough breads

Vinegar (except white vinegar) found in:

Relishes

Catsup

Mustard

Salad dressing

Worcestershire sauce

Steak sauce

Chili sauce

Nuts and peanut butter

Potatoes

Seeds

Sunflower

Pumpkin

Sesame

Coffee

Nitrites found in:

Hot dogs

Bologna

Bacon	Sausage
Ham	Pepperoni
Salami	

Sugar substitute

Aspartame

Monosodium glutamate (MSG) found in:

Chinese foods	Dry roasted nuts
Instant rice	Instant gravies
Soup	Potato chips
TV dinners	Meat tenderizers and seasonings

Miscellaneous

| Soy products (bean curd, miso soup) | Sodium benzoate |
| Licorice | Garlic |

If you find that one of the foods on this list triggers a migraine, then all of these foods are suspect. For example, if chocolate is a migraine trigger, then you may well find citrus, cheese and the other foods in Table 3.1 to be migraine triggers. Sometimes two triggers must be combined for a migraine to result. Cheese alone might not trigger a headache, but it could produce a migraine if combined with another trigger.

Such alcoholic beverages as red wine, beer, and sherry trigger headaches. Alcoholic beverages less likely to provoke a headache include white wine, rum, scotch, and vodka. The kind of headache I am referring to is a migraine resulting from serotonin-provoked vasodilation and should not be confused with the hangover headache that results several hours after drinking has stopped. The hangover headache is a withdrawal symptom and has nothing to do with migraine. It happens to anyone who has consumed too much alcohol.

As a vasoconstrictor, caffeine can help reduce the pain of a migraine attack. However, more than 200 mg of caffeine can produce a caffeine withdrawal headache. There are two ways to handle caffeine. One is to keep your intake at a steady state so that withdrawal does not take place. Using this approach, no more than 12 hours should elapse without caffeine. The second approach is to reduce your intake of caffeine so that it does not exceed 200 mg daily. This amount includes the caffeine in coffee, tea, soda, and in such medications as aspirin and various ergot preparations. The median amount of caffeine in coffee and tea is listed in Table 3.2.

Table 3.2
Caffeine Content of Coffee and Tea

Brewed coffee/cup	100 mg[1]
Instant coffee/cup	85 mg
Tea/cup	70 mg

If you decide to give up coffee and tea altogether, do so gradually. I experienced one of my worse migraines when I stopped my consumption of coffee abruptly.

Add up the caffeine in the coffee and tea you drink each day. Add to this figure the caffeine in any medications you might be taking (see Tables 2.1 and 2.2), the caffeine in the aspirin you take (which is listed on the label), and the caffeine in your soft drinks. The total amount might surprise you.

Serotonin is an amine made in the body from dietary tryptophan. Turkey contains tryptophan. As we learned earlier, altered serotonin levels can trigger vasodilation and headache. I have found turkey, because of its relationship to serotonin, to be a migraine trigger.

The preservative benozoic acid and the yellow dye tartrazine (FD & C No. 5) have been reported to cause headaches in some people. Children seem especially susceptible to these food additives. Sodium benzoate, which I have found to be a migraine trigger, is the sodium salt of benzoic acid. Benzoic acid occurs naturally in such foods as cranberries, raspberries, prunes, cinnamon, plums, and ripe olives. After eating a snack of cinnamon toast one evening, I awoke in the morning with a terrible migraine. I now know the headache was caused by the benzoic acid in the cinnamon.

---

1. These figures represent an average.

Low blood sugar can cause migraine headaches because this condition starts a chemical chain reaction that results in dilated cerebral blood vessels. In some people, refined sugar stimulates the pancreas to release excess insulin that metabolizes not only the sugar just eaten but also any sugar already present in the bloodstream. The result is a lower blood sugar level than before the sugar was eaten. By avoiding sugar altogether, this process of rapid rise/rapid fall in blood sugar levels does not take place, thus preventing a migraine from developing.

If all refined sugar is avoided, where does the body get its energy? The natural sugar in fresh fruit and unsweetened fruit juice does not trigger the insulin chain reaction outlined above. Another source is such carbohydrates as rice, bread, and pasta. Some carbohydrates should be eaten with each meal to offset the lack of refined sugar in the diet.

Avoiding sugar did not help my migraines, nor is it mentioned in the scientific literature as a migraine trigger. I include it here because I have read a few case histories in which the migraineur was helped when he or she stopped eating refined sugar. It is very likely that in these cases, blood sugar levels fell because a sugar snack *replaced* a balanced meal. When a dessert containing sugar *follows* a balanced meal, a migraine attack is not usually triggered.

The sugar level in the blood also decreases when too much time has elapsed between meals. Some migraine sufferers have found that if they eat every four hours their headaches disappear. A protein snack at bedtime will often prevent a morning headache. I have found, for example, that I can sometimes eliminate morning migraines by having a sandwich before going to bed.

If your blood sugar is abnormally low, you might have a condition called hypoglycemia. Your doctor can determine if you are hypoglycemic by giving you a glucose tolerance test. Symptoms of hypoglycemia include lightheadedness, sweating, and headache. Even if you are not hypoglycemic, headache can result if you do not have something to eat every four hours. Many migraine sufferers have had their headaches totally stop when they ate every four hours and had a protein snack at bedtime.

I avoid all of the amine-containing foods listed in Table 3.1. The few times I have cheated and eaten one of these foods, a headache has usually followed. I was able to see what other foods might trigger a headache by eliminating all foods for up to five days except those with no headache-causing potential (Table 3.3). At the end of this period, I reintroduced foods one at a time to my diet. If a headache developed, I knew that food would have to be eliminated. I also ate bedtime and between meal snacks from Table 3.3 so that no more than four hours would elapse without some food intake during waking hours. Headaches may get worse before improving during this testing period.

Table 3.3
Foods With No Known Headache Causing Potential

Meat

Lamb	Chicken

Fruit

Pears	Unsweetened pear juice

Vegetables

Brussel sprouts	Carrots
Zucchini	Broccoli
Cauliflower	

After adding back a fair amount of foods, I found that eggs and milk were headache triggers for me. When I avoided these foods, amine-containing foods, nitrites, MSG, sodium benzoate, and the sugar substitute aspartame, my headaches decreased considerably. For the first time in eight months, I had headache-free periods that lasted for days.

In summary, many migraine sufferers have to accept the fact that they cannot eat foods containing amines if they want to become headache free. It should be noted that upon occasion a small amount of amine-containing foods can be tolerated; but once we go over a certain critical level, headache results. Since we cannot always predict what this level is, it is best to avoid these foods altogether. In addition, do not skip meals. The foods you eat are powerful migraine triggers and many headaches can be avoided by alterations in the diet.

4

Nondietary Migraine Triggers

In addition to diet, migraine triggers include stress, sleep, altitude, chemicals, medicines, vitamins, weather, flickering light, exercise, and sex.

Research has shown that migraineurs are not more sensitive to stress than nonmigraineurs. Some migraine authorities suggest that stress releases serotonin. It is the reaction to serotonin, and not a particular susceptibility to stress, that causes the headache. Some migraineurs get their headaches during the let down period following the stressful situation when serotonin levels are falling.

Discussing stress as a migraine trigger is a complicated issue because it implies that migraine sufferers are overly sensitive people who cannot handle stress properly. This is simply not the case. Until approximately ten years ago, migraine sufferers were thought to be obsessive, perfectionist, driven people. Personality tests given since that time show that the personality traits of migraineurs do not differ from those of the general population. Migraine sufferers do not have unique personalities that would predispose them to be particularly sensitive to stress. I prefer to think of migraineurs as people in whom stress sets up a biochemical alteration that produces headache. It is this constitutional biochemical process, and not environmental stress per se, that triggers the migraine attack.

Excessive or too little sleep may also precipitate a migraine. Sleeping late over the weekend is a common cause of headaches. It is best to get up at the same time each day, including weekends.

Vasodilation at altitudes above 8000 feet, brought about by a reduction in oxygen, can cause headaches. I remember camping in the Sierra Nevada mountains many years ago. I was feeling fine until I had a glass of red wine while sitting around the campfire. The combination of the two triggers—altitude and red wine—resulted in a terrible migraine.

A variety of chemicals, including carbon tetrachloride, benzene, insecticides, and home insulation products made from formaldehyde, have been reported to cause headaches. Strong smells, a smoke-filled room, or a poorly ventilated room may trigger a headache. Carbon monoxide can be a migraine trigger. Some people report less frequent and less intense headaches when they stop smoking. This may be because carbon monoxide is present in cigarette smoke. Smokers have been found to have a higher blood level of carbon monoxide than nonsmokers.

Some medicines can trigger a migraine. Nitroglycerin is used to treat heart disease and has been known to cause migraines. Other migraine triggers include lithium, the antihypertensive drugs reserpine and hydralazine, the anti-inflammatory drug indomethacin, diuretics, and the bronchodilating drug Aminophylline and the other theophyllines. If you get migraines and are taking any of these drugs, you should ask your doctor to change your prescription.

Sinus and cold medications may trigger headaches. I would be wary of any compounds containing ephedrine (a decongestant), chlorpheniramine maleate (an antihistamine), or phenylpropanolamine (a decongestant). A chemical that has "amine" as part of its name should be avoided. I recently bought a cold medication that promised relief without drowsiness. Not containing antihistamines, I thought this drug would be safe. The next morning I had a cold that was now accompanied by a migraine. I read the label only to discover this medication contained the migraine trigger ephedrine.

Withdrawal headaches from aspirin, acetaminophen, and ergotamine occur with daily use of these drugs. More of the drug is then taken to combat the withdrawal headache. A cycle is established that leads to chronic daily headaches and dependence on these drugs to relieve the headache that they have caused. More than 1000 mg of aspirin or acetaminophen must be taken daily in order for withdrawal headaches to occur.

A chronic headache sufferer can easily exceed 1000 mg of aspirin or acetaminophen each day. For example, in order to combat a particularly bad migraine, I had taken three Tylenol tablets and two Midrin capsules in the course of one day for a total of 1625 mg of acetaminophen. A withdrawal headache followed, which I could have treated with more Tylenol and Midrin. If I had done so, my headache would have become chronic, and dependency on these drugs would have ensued.

Some migraine patients do not even think of aspirin or Tylenol as drugs. They take them much as they might take vitamins. Taking two or three aspirin or Tylenol each morning might have become a life-long habit. According to some migraine authorities, daily headaches are withdrawal symptoms from the chronic use of ergotamine, aspirin, or acetaminophen. Stopping such chronic use is very hard and may require hospitalization. One way to break the habit is to taper off of these drugs by taking less each day. Another way is to stop their use abruptly. You may experience a headache for from three to seven days before the headache disappears entirely. If you have stopped all of the triggers listed in this book and your headache continues on a daily basis, chances are it is caused by one or more of the medications you are taking.

Antianxiety drugs, such as Librium and Valium, serve no purpose in the treatment of migraine. Even a small amount of these drugs can cause withdrawal headaches. If your doctor has prescribed an antianxiety drug for your migraines, please get a second opinion about your need for this medication.

Even vitamin pills are not as benign as we once thought. From 25,000 to 50,000 IU of vitamin A may trigger a headache. If you eat foods that are high in vitamin A, such as carrots, and take a supplement with 25,000 IU of A, you would be over your limit, and a headache could result. Large doses of niacin (nicotinic acid) can also trigger a migraine. Nicotinic acid is a vasodilator and should only be taken during the aura phase in classic migraine.

Many vitamins contain such migraine triggers as yeast, citrus, and soy. If you must take vitamins, you might want to take one of the hypo-allergenic brands that avoid these substances. I have found many vitamin pills to be migraine triggers.

I have also found that one 600 mg tablet of calcium is safe, while two 600 mg tablets of calcium per day will trigger a headache. It is not the calcium, but rather the other ingredients that the manufacturers put in the pills that are the headache triggers. At the present time, I am experimenting with calcium made from oyster shells, since it is a pure substance with no added ingredients.

Weather conditions can precipitate a migraine attack. Wind, a thunderstorm, the sun's glare on snow or water, and very cold temperatures or high humidity are migraine triggers for some people. I am particularly sensitive to strong sunlight on a hot day. If I do not wear a hat and sunglasses at the beach, the heat and glare of the sun will trigger a headache.

Some people find that the flickering light from a television or movie screen or the flicker from fluorescent lights will trigger a headache. Wearing sunglasses or tinted lenses may help this condition.

Exercise can also be a migraine trigger, especially vigorous exercise by people not physically fit. Exercise headaches can reflect a serious medical problem. You should see your doctor if you get headaches while exercising.

The orgasmic headache, most common in men, is a form of effort headache that occurs during orgasm. Like the exercise headache, orgasmic headaches may indicate a serious underlying condition and should be discussed with your doctor.

Nondietary migraine triggers are listed in Table 4.1.

Table 4.1

Nondietary Migraine Triggers

Stress

Sleep

Excessive	Fatigue

Altitude

Chemicals

Carbon tetrachloride	Benzene
Insecticides	Formaldehyde
Carbon monoxide	

Environment

Strong smells	Smoke
Poor ventilation	Flickering light

Medicines

Nitroglycerin	Hydralazine
Lithium	Reserpine
Indomethacin	Diuretics
Antihistamines	Aspirin
Acetaminophen	Ergotamine
Librium, Valium	Decongestants with
Theophyllines	phenylpropanolamine or
(Aminophylline)	ephedrine

Vitamins

Vitamin A	Niacin

Weather

Wind	Thunderstorms
Glare	Cold temperatures
High humidity	

Exercise

Sex

In summary, a variety of environmental conditions and nondietary substances can trigger a migraine. I would suggest paying particular attention to your sleep patterns. Try not to get too much or too little sleep. Also, to avoid withdrawal headaches, take less than 1000 mg of aspirin or Tylenol daily and do not use ergotamine medications every day.

5

Headache as a Symptom of Disease

A basic question must be asked about any migraine headache. Is it a disease in and of itself, or is it a symptom of an underlying disorder? This question is especially important if migraine attacks have just begun or if ongoing migraines change in their frequency, intensity, or characteristics. The computed axiel tomography (CAT) scan or magnetic resonance imaging (MRI) and blood tests are routinely given to determine the cause of the headache. Depending on symptoms, an angiogram, lumbar puncture, or other tests might also be called for.

A brain tumor is something that all headache patients fear. A CAT scan or MRI takes X-ray type pictures of the brain that show the presence of a tumor. Brain tumors are very rare but their possibility must be ruled out immediately.

Sixty percent of the people who have brain tumors will have a headache. In the majority of these cases, the pain is dull, nonthrobbing, and intermittent. It may be made worse by changing positions or coughing. The headache may be accompanied by loss of smell or hearing, personality changes, alterations in vision, loss of balance, and weakness or numbness in one-half of the body. Approximately 50 percent of people with brain tumors experience nausea and vomiting.

A hemorrhage from a ruptured aneurysm produces a violent, continuous headache, which may be accompanied by vomiting, a stiff neck, drowsiness, and loss of consciousness. The headache comes suddenly and is sometimes described as feeling like an explosion. A CAT scan or MRI will reveal a ruptured aneurysm. An unruptured aneurysm may also be signaled by a headache described as similar to an explosion or a clap of thunder. An angiogram is used to locate the unruptured aneurysm.

Infections are a common cause of headache. The presence of many infections can be determined by blood tests.

Daily headache may be one of the symptoms of the Epstein-Barr virus. Other symptoms include malaise, fatigue, lymph node enlargement, fever, and a sore throat. In some cases, headache and fatigue continue after other symptoms cease to exist.

Lyme disease is an infection transmitted by mouse or deer ticks. In addition to headache, Lyme disease may produce malaise, fatigue, arthritis-like symptoms, stiff neck, muscular pain, and fever. If untreated, neurological abnormalities may develop.

Meningitis is an infection that causes headache, fever, neck stiffness, seizures, vomiting, and an aversion to bright light. It is an inflammation of the covering of the brain, the meninges, which is usually produced by a viral or bacterial infection.

Unlike viral meningitis, bacterial meningitis can be life-threatening. The infecting agent gains entry into the brain through the nose, sinuses, ear, or bloodstream. The diagnosis of meningitis can be confirmed by an examination of spinal fluid that is removed by lumbar puncture.

Other infections accompanied by headache include tonsillitis, pneumonia, scarlet fever, typhoid fever, typhus fever, influenza, smallpox, rabies, mumps, measles, herpes simplex, poliomyelitis, and malaria. In most cases, the headache disappears when the infection subsides.

Multiple sclerosis is another serious disease that is accompanied by head pain in a minority of cases. MRI and spinal fluid examination are good diagnostic indicators of this disease. Symptoms of multiple sclerosis may include spasticity, tremor, disturbances of speech, ocular movements, impaired vision, bladder problems, and weakness, numbness, or paralysis in one or more extremity.

The mouth and eyes can also be the source of headaches. Abscesses in the mouth and cracked teeth can lead to head pain that may resemble migraine. If you have headaches, a checkup by your dentist is in order.

Eye strain as well as a rare form of glaucoma can cause headaches. An eye examination by an ophthalmologist will disclose the presence of these conditions.

Systemic lupus erythematosus, giant cell arteritis (or temporal arteritis, as it is sometimes called), and polymyalgia rheumatica are three inflammatory diseases that often include headache as one of their symptoms.

Lupus is a disease that damages the connective tissue throughout the body. Inflammation of the membranes surrounding the kidneys, lungs, joints, and other organs is common. In addition to headaches, a few of the many symptoms of lupus are fever, muscle pain, fatigue, anemia, weight loss, joint pain, hair loss, and sometimes a red rash on the face and other areas exposed to the sun. Blood tests will confirm a diagnosis of lupus.

Giant cell arteritis is an inflammatory disease of the arteries of the temples that usually develops in people over 50 years of age. The headache that accompanies this disorder is a dull ache that may be sharp at times on one or both sides of the head. The pain is described as having a burning quality. There may be tenderness or swelling of the temporal artery. The pain itself may radiate to this artery. The headache is often slightly worse at night. Muscular aches and pains, weight loss, low-grade fever, fatigue, scalp tenderness, and jaw claudication, or pain when chewing, are symptomatic of the disease. If not treated, giant cell arteritis can lead to blindness and stroke. Blood tests may show an elevated sedimentation rate, abnormal liver function, and anemia. The diagnosis of giant cell arteritis can be confirmed by a biopsy of the temporal artery.

Polymyalgia rheumatica is caused by an inflammation of the muscles. It is characterized by muscle aches in the neck, shoulders, and hips. It usually does not affect people under 50 years of age. Other symptoms include headache, morning stiffness, fatigue, weight loss and a low-grade fever. Some people think polymyalgia rheumatica and giant cell arteritis represent different stages in the same disease process. Blood test abnormalities are similar in both diseases.

Many people who have a heart malfunction known as mitral valve prolapse also suffer from headaches. Other symptoms of this condition include fatigue, chest pain, palpitations, and dizziness. Platelet aggregation on the abnormal valve may play a role in the development of headache. Echocardiography is used to confirm the diagnosis of mitral valve prolapse.

Cushing's syndrome is a disorder resulting from increased production of cortisol by the adrenal gland. Elevated cortisol levels can be caused by an adrenal tumor, a pituitary tumor, or prolonged use of steroid medications. Approximately one-half of the patients with this syndrome experience headaches. In addition, fatigue, muscle weakness, osteoporosis, obesity, hypertension, a "moon face," and, in women, cessation of menses and excessive face and body hair are common symptoms of the disease. The diagnosis of Cushing's syndrome is based on the results of a dexamethasone-suppression test.

Anywhere from 30 to 80 percent of head injury patients experience headaches. The headache that results from a concussion may be either dull or throbbing in nature. Movement of the head or body may worsen the headache. It may be accompanied by amnesia, irritability, nausea, vomiting, vertigo, or difficulty in concentration. The headache may develop days or weeks after the injury and can last from days to years. Headache also commonly follows whiplash injuries, along with vertigo, dizziness, ringing in the ears, and visual disturbances. In addition, some people experience mood changes, anxiety, difficulties in thinking, and insomnia following an injury to the head. X-rays may be required after a concussion to detect a possible fracture. A CAT scan might be necessary to rule out hemorrhage following a severe blow to the head.

Common disorders accompanied by headache, along with their diagnostic tests, are listed in Table 5.1. Uncommon causes of headaches include very high blood pressure, cervical spine disease, a jaw disorder called temporomandibular joint (TMJ) dysfunction, constipation, and sinus disease.

The headache caused by high blood pressure is usually experienced as pain in the back of the head and neck. The blood pressure must be severely elevated in order to produce head pain. In some cases, it is the medication used to treat high blood pressure that is the cause of the headache.

In cervical spine disease, rheumatoid arthritis and nerve root entrapment due to osteoarthritic changes in the cervical spine can cause pain in the neck and back of the head that sometimes radiates to the forehead. Most of the neck pain experienced by headache sufferers, however, stems from conditions other than cervical spine disease. The majority of people with rheumatoid arthritis or degenerative diseases of the spine do not have chronic headaches.

Head pain from TMJ dysfunction originates in the jaw and can radiate to the ear and temple. A click in the jaw when chewing or talking may indicate the presence of this condition. The pain is thought to be due to muscle spasms resulting from grinding or clenching the teeth or from an uneven bite. Many professionals feel that the connection between TMJ dysfunction and headache has been exaggerated.

Headache resulting from constipation is a controversial issue. Some experts feel that accumulated toxins or an expanded bowel can precipitate a headache. Other authorities see no connection between headache and constipation.

You might wonder why sinus disease is listed as an "uncommon" cause of headaches. Pain results when the sinuses become filled with fluid as a result of infection, tumors, or allergic reactions. These conditions are rare and many so-called sinus headaches are in reality muscle contraction or migraine headaches. X-rays will indicate the presence of sinus disease.

The removal of spinal fluid during lumbar puncture may cause a headache of short duration. Lying down and drinking fluids helps relieve the headache. As soon as spinal fluid pressure returns to normal, the pain disappears.

Table 5.1

Common Disorders Accompanied by Headache

DISORDER	TEST
Brain tumor	MRI or CAT scan
Aneurysm	
Ruptured	MRI or CAT scan
Unruptured	Angiogram
Infections[1]	
Epstein-Barr	Blood test
Lyme disease	Blood test
Meningitis	Lumbar puncture
Multiple sclerosis	MRI, lumbar puncture
Mouth	
Abscesses	Dental exam

1. Most infections are accompanied by headache. See text for a complete list.

DISORDER	TEST
Cracked teeth	Dental exam
Eyes	
Eye strain	Eye exam
Glaucoma	Eye exam
Systemic lupus erythematosus (SLE)	Blood test
Giant cell arteritis	Blood test, Biopsy of temporal artery
Polymyalgia rheumatica	Blood test
Mitral valve prolapse	Echocardiogram
Cushing's syndrome	Dexamethasone-suppression test
Head injuries	
Concussion	Depends on severity of injury
Whiplash	

Many neuralgias causing facial pain are beyond the scope of this book. They have distinctive pain patterns and are seldom mistaken for migraine.

I have had a MRI, an echocardiogram, a dental exam, an eye exam, and a variety of blood tests. Because my symptoms did not include a fever, I was not tested for meningitis. All of my tests were negative. It is important to note that you could test positive for one of these conditions and not have all of the symptoms listed in the chapter.

In summary, it would be wise to have a complete physical examination, including a CAT scan or MRI, to rule out headache as a symptom of an underlying disorder. This is especially true if your headaches are new or have changed in their frequency, intensity, or characteristics.

6

Hormones and Migraine

As many as 60 percent of the women prone to migraine find that their headaches intensify just prior to, during, or immediately after menstruation. Decreasing estrogen levels seem to play a role in the migraines experienced during this period. One theory holds that estrogen controls the release of serotonin. As estrogen levels fall, serotonin decreases and vasodilation results.

Anaprox (naproxen), Inderal (propranolol), and various ergotamine preparations are the more common medications used in the treatment of menstrual migraine. However, these drugs, as well as the other medications discussed in chapter 2, have limited success in preventing headaches associated with menstruation. Ponstel (mefenamic acid) is a nonsteroidal anti-inflammatory drug, not discussed in chapter 2, that is used to treat menstrual migraine. Danocrine (danazol), a synthetic androgen, has also been used with some success in the treatment of migraine associated with menstruation. Prophylactic migraine medications are usually begun three days before menses begins and are continued throughout the period of menstruation.

More than 70 percent of female migraine sufferers find that their headaches improve during the second and third trimester of pregnancy only to return after delivery. Some women experience migraines for the first time following delivery. A minority of women who have had migraines all of their lives find that their headaches worsen during pregnancy.

Some researchers feel that high estrogen and progesterone levels during the second and third trimester account for the decrease in migraines. Other researchers stress the correlation between low headache levels and increased production of endorphins during these months. Endorphins are called the body's natural pain killers because of their narcotic-like properties.

Most drugs that treat or prevent migraines cannot be taken by pregnant women for fear they will harm the fetus. One headache authority feels that Demerol (meperidine) is a safe migraine medication that can be taken during pregnancy if it is not taken every day and if daily doses do not exceed 400 mg.[1] Tylenol (acetaminophen) is also considered safe by most physicians. Many feel that aspirin, on the other hand, should be avoided by pregnant women. If you have migraines and are pregnant, check with your doctor before taking any headache medications. Fortunately, headaches usually disappear after the first trimester, and medication will not be needed after that period.

You might think that synthetic estrogen and progesterone added to a woman's natural supply of these hormones would decrease migraines much as an overabundance of hormones decreases headaches during pregnancy. Such is not the case with the birth control pill. Some women experience migraines for the first time while taking "the pill." Fifty percent of migraine sufferers who take oral contraceptives find that their headaches increase in intensity. As can be expected with the serendipity of this disorder, a small number of women find their headaches improve when they take birth control pills.

For most women with pre-existing migraine, headaches occur during the week between cycles when the pill is stopped and hormone levels fall. Women who had migraines for the first time while taking birth control pills do not fall into this pattern. In addition, migraine sufferers, especially those with classic migraine, increase their risk of stroke and other blood vessel disorders when taking oral contraceptives. If you are subject to migraines, birth control pills should be replaced with other forms of contraception.

---

1. Raskin, N.H. (1988): *Headache*. New York: Churchill Livingstone, p. 155.

As estrogen and progesterone decrease during menopause, some women begin to experience migraines for the first time. Almost 50 percent of migraine sufferers find that their headaches worsen when their menstrual cycles stop. Paradoxically, in a minority of women, headaches decrease or stop altogether during menopause. In many cases, estrogen replacement therapy (ERT) tends to intensify pre-existing migraines. However, a small minority of women found that ERT helped their headaches. In these cases, synthetic estrogen was more beneficial than estrogen derived from animal sources.

Three years after beginning menopause, I began to experience daily headaches. I thought that ERT would replicate my pre-menopausal hormonal environment and I would only get migraines during the phase in the monthly cycle when synthetic estrogen was stopped. During the six months I was on ERT, and contrary to all logic, my headaches not only continued on a daily basis, they actually increased in intensity. Perhaps my experience would have been different if I had tried the noncyclic method in which a small amount of estrogen and progesterone is taken each day in the month with no break.

Why does a drop in estrogen cause headaches during menstruation and menopause? One theory, discussed at the beginning of this chapter, stresses the fact that serotonin is controlled by falling estrogen levels. As serotonin levels decline, blood vessels in the brain dilate producing headache.

Why would increased amounts of estrogen due to ERT or the birth control pill cause headaches? Examination of the endometrial tissue of women taking oral contraceptives has shown an increase in monoamine oxidase (MAO). MAO is an enzyme that metabolizes serotonin. Reduced serotonin levels can cause vasodilation and headache.

In summary, it appears that whenever estrogen is either increased synthetically, as in ERT or the contraceptive pill, or decreased dramatically, as in menstruation or menopause, headache often results. Scientific investigation has provided us with little proof as to how altered estrogen levels produce headaches. At this point the connection between estrogen and migraines is purely speculative.

7

Mixed Headaches

Many people experience both migraine and muscle contraction, or tension, headaches. What is the difference between these two types of headache? Muscle contraction headaches are commonly thought to arise from a state of tension in the body. When the body is tense, muscles in the head and neck contract, thus giving rise to pain. Migraine, on the other hand, seems to come from a chemical alteration in the body that leads to dilated blood vessels.

Muscle contraction headaches may be either acute or chronic. Chronic muscle contraction headaches may occur daily or almost daily. In mixed headaches, migraine is superimposed upon, or alternates with, the muscle contraction headache. Sometimes the muscle contraction component of the mixed headache syndrome is, in fact, a rebound headache caused by daily use of analgesics or ergotamine. Over 1000 mg of aspirin or acetaminophen (Tylenol) taken on a daily basis can cause chronic rebound headaches.

Muscle contraction headaches may be experienced as a tight band around the head that can radiate into the neck and shoulders. The pain is usually felt on both sides of the head, whereas the pain in migraine is commonly on one side only. The pain is often dull and constant. It does not pulsate as in a migraine headache. Visual abnormalities and nausea or vomiting do not usually accompany muscle contraction headaches.

Muscle contraction headaches may be a symptom of depression as well as emotional stress. Frustration has been known to trigger a muscle contraction headache. Sometimes these headaches have a purely physical cause, such as sitting hunched over a typewriter or word processor for a long period of time.

Some people may react in a psychologically normal fashion to stressful situations, but their muscles, for reasons unknown to medical science, contract in such a way that headache results. When stressed, all animals, including humans, experience a fight or flight reaction. Muscles contract in preparation for fight or flight. Why in some cases such muscle contraction is accompanied by headache and in other cases it is not is unknown.

In migraine headaches, pain results from the dilation of blood vessels in the brain. In contrast, the pain in muscle contraction headaches is caused by muscles that are in a state of contraction or spasm. Blood vessels have been found to be constricted during headache periods.

Muscle contraction headaches that occur infrequently, say once or twice a month, can usually be treated with aspirin. If stronger medication is needed, Fiorinal tablets or capsules have been successful in eliminating the pain associated with these headaches. Fiorinal, with or without codeine, is composed of aspirin, caffeine, and butalbital, a barbiturate. Butalbital has muscle relaxant properties that make it particularly effective in treating muscle contraction headaches.

I have found exercise to be helpful in eliminating my infrequent muscle contraction headaches. The following three exercises will reduce neck and shoulder tension:

1.   Lay on your back on a carpeted floor with your knees flexed and arms at your sides. Raise your shoulders up toward your ears then return to starting position. Repeat ten times.

2.   Lay on your back on a carpeted floor with your knees flexed. Alternately raise each arm straight back until the back of your finger tips touch the floor, maintaining a continuous motion. Repeat each cycle fifteen times.

3.   Lay on your back on a carpeted floor with knees flexed. Rest hands on your stomach. Turn your head as far to the left as you can. Return to center and then turn your head as far as you can to the right. Repeat each cycle fifteen times or until neck muscles no longer pull.

Wet heat in the form of a damp washcloth on top of a heating pad applied to the back of the neck is another method of reducing the pain of muscle contraction headaches.

If muscle contraction headaches occur frequently, a concerted effort might have to be made to investigate methods of achieving relaxation. In addition, you might want to explore the possibility of taking antidepressant medication. Even if you are not depressed, a small dose of antidepressant medication (perhaps as little as 10 mg) may be helpful in muscle contraction headaches as well as migraine. In difficult cases, a beta blocking drug, such as Inderal, may be combined with the antidepressant.

Antianxiety drugs such as Valium (diazepam), Librium (chlordiazepoxide) or Miltown (meprobamate) are to be avoided since they only treat symptoms and do nothing to help you eliminate the cause of your tension or anxiety. In addition, antianxiety drugs, or tranquilizers, are addicting in that you need increased doses of the drug to be effective, and withdrawal symptoms are experienced if they are stopped abruptly. These drugs have been known to cause rebound headaches in migraine sufferers.

Biofeedback has shown good results in reducing the pain of muscle contraction headaches. The goal of this treatment is to learn to control muscle tension through mental imaging. Biofeedback is discussed in detail in chapter 8. Muscle contraction headaches have also been helped by the relaxation that results from daily meditation, yoga, massage, and exercise.

In summary, if muscle contraction headaches are a chronic condition, methods of reducing tension must be investigated. The possibility of depression should be explored. If muscle contraction headaches are infrequent, a drug such as Fiorinal might be of help. People who get frequent mixed headaches might benefit from antidepressant medication.

8

Biofeedback and Other Alternatives

For centuries, Eastern practitioners have been able to control involuntary body processes with the mind. Anyone who has visited India and watched holy men walking barefoot over burning coals will attest to the possibility of such control. Blood pressure, heart rate, muscle tension, and skin temperature are functions of the autonomic nervous system that can be regulated by mental imagery using a technique known as biofeedback.

Biofeedback teaches thought control over body processes by a system of reinforcement. An electromyographic (EMG) monitor measures muscle tension. A visual or auditory signal indicates when relaxation has achieved a reduction in muscle tension. The desired result is reinforced until muscle tension comes under voluntary control. At this point the EMG monitor is no longer needed. Any technique that reduces muscle tension holds promise in the treatment of muscle contraction headaches.

Vascular, or migraine, headaches have been successfully treated by increasing hand temperature. In this case, a thermistor is taped to the subject's finger to measure skin temperature. This device indicates when thought processes have been successful in increasing hand temperature. The process is reinforced until hand warming can be achieved by voluntary control. As the arteries in the hand dilate, it is believed that those in the head will constrict, thus relieving pain caused by dilated cranial blood vessels. Biofeedback has been most successful in people with classic migraine. In these cases, the headache is aborted during the aura phase before the pain itself is experienced.

One drawback of biofeedback is that the relaxation exercises must be practiced at home every day. The goal of stopping pharmacological treatment, with its unpleasant side effects, is motivation enough for many headache sufferers to try to master this technique. For some people, biofeedback used along with pharmacological therapy allows a reduction in the amount of the drug being used.

Does biofeedback work? Results are mixed. Some researchers have found that relaxation exercises alone are as effective as biofeedback for muscle contraction headaches. In other studies, from 39 to 50 percent of the subjects felt both migraines and muscle contraction headaches had improved. In yet another study, 87 percent experienced improvement. A fewer number of migraine sufferers were able to eradicate their headaches completely when using biofeedback. Nevertheless, any improvement in headache intensity and duration that might allow a reduction in drug use would be of value.

If you want to try biofeedback, it is important that you go to a facility where a professional trained in biofeedback is on staff. If your physician or headache clinic does not offer this modality, ask them to refer you to a pain clinic in your area. Biofeedback is one of the treatment procedures offered by many pain clinics. Be sure the instructor understands that different approaches are used for migraine and muscle contraction headaches. As a migraine sufferer, you will want to learn the hand warming technique. If you have both migraines and muscle contraction headaches, you will also want to learn the muscle tension reduction technique.

Acupuncture is another nondrug modality that has been used to treat migraine. It is an ancient Chinese method of medical treatment in which very fine needles are inserted in the body on specially designated points along what are called meridians. Some practitioners use a battery or electrically powered device to provide electrical stimulation through the needles.

Acupuncture is regarded by many as less effective than biofeedback in migraine treatment. Some improvement might be experienced due to the release of the body's natural painkillers known as endorphins. Studies have shown that over time improvement is temporary. Although acupuncture is a common treatment for headaches in China, Western researchers are less enthusiastic about its long-term benefit for migraine sufferers. Perhaps results in the West are often negative because so many unqualified people are administering this technique. J.N. Blau makes this point in the following quote from a paper by C.A. Vincent and P.H. Richardson.[1]

> To a traditional acupuncturist most of the acupuncture practiced in the west is akin to an unqualified person handing out antibiotics at random to sick people. The traditional healer utilizes subtle signs in diagnosis including pulses, the complexion and smell of the patient, whereas trigger points, tender areas, points in the same dermatome as the pain, have little in common with traditional acupuncture other than the insertion of needles.

If you want to try acupuncture, be sure you go to a certified practitioner. The training of practitioners is discussed in a comparison of Eastern and Western acupuncture in chapter 14.

Chiropractic therapy offers little help for the migraine sufferer. Chiropractors view disease as stemming from displaced vertebrae that disrupt nerve functioning. Nerve interference can also take place in the muscles and joints. According to chiropractic theory, relieving the pressure on the nerves through manipulation or massage cures certain diseases.

I could find no studies in which chiropractic techniques were shown to abort or prevent migraine headaches. Gentle neck massage may help to relieve muscle contraction headaches. Vigorous manipulation of the neck and spine, however, can be extremely dangerous and should be avoided.

Trager Mentastics is another modality that makes use of the mind-body continuum to relieve pain. The dance-like movements of this approach produce relaxation and a meditative state that serve as a preventative treatment for muscle contraction headaches and for the tension headache component that accompanies migraine in the mixed headache syndrome. Trager Mentastics can be done at home. Trager Psychophysical Integration, on the other hand, is a form of hands-on bodywork done by skilled practitioners.[2] Jan

---

1. Vincent, C.A. and Richardson, P.H. (1986): The evaluation of therapeutic acupuncture: Concepts and methods. *Pain* 24: 1-13. Reprinted in Blau, J.N., ed. (1987): *Migraine: Clinical and Research Aspects.* Baltimore: The Johns Hopkins University Press.
2. A list of certified Trager practitioners in your area can be obtained by writing to: The Trager Institute, 10 Old Mill Street, Mill Valley, California 94941.

Bennett, Trager practitioner at the Neurologic Centre for Headache and Pain in La Jolla, California, describes this modality as follows:

With the patient lying on the treatment table the practitioner lifts each body part and with gentle rocking, stretching, compression, and rotation movements encourages the muscles to let go. The practitioner nonverbally supports the patient to experience and incorporate the sensation of muscular lightness and freedom of movement. Trager Psychophysical Integration achieves more lasting results than more traditional methods because the muscle groups are handled in rhythmic, rocking, and stretching motions that prevent both the development of resistance and the return to habitual patterns of tension.

Pain clinics are beginning to realize the importance of body-mind interaction in headache treatment. For example, at the Neurologic Centre for Headache and Pain in La Jolla, California, Trager bodywork is a standard treatment for clients who suffer from tension headaches or migraines with a muscle contraction component. Other modalities used to treat headaches at this facility include medication, psychotherapy, chiropractic treatment, and biofeedback. Chiropractic therapy is used to treat the headache that may result form neck injuries, such as the whiplash injuries associated with automobile accidents. As far as migraine treatment is concerned, Dr. David Hubbard, director of the center, says that they have had the most success with biofeedback. Patients have been found to achieve an 87 percent reduction in the frequency and severity of their migraines in an average of 14 sessions of biofeedback. Trager bodywork is combined with biofeedback if the migraine patient also suffers from tension headaches.

In summary, of the techniques discussed in this chapter, biofeedback holds the most promise for migraine sufferers. If diet and lifestyle changes do not reduce your migraines, biofeedback might be worth exploring. At most, you may be able to abort or prevent your migraines using biofeedback. At the very least, your headaches may be reduced in intensity and duration.

9

Finding the Right Doctor

You have every right to have your headaches taken seriously by your doctor. If he or she implies you are neurotic or tells you your headaches are caused by "nerves," go to another doctor immediately. If he or she wants to treat your migraine headaches with tranquilizers, get another opinion.

Most doctors who specialize in the treatment of migraine are neurologists; however, not all neurologists have the sensitivity, training, or patience to be right for you. You may have to shop around. In the United States, you may want to call the National Headache Foundation in Chicago at 1-800-843-2256 (in Illinois the number is 1-800-523-8858) for a list of physicians in your area who belong to the foundation.

The Migraine Foundation of Canada cannot give the public its membership list of headache specialists. The Canadian Medical Association will only allow this information to be released to physicians. If you live in Canada, ask your doctor to call the Migraine Foundation of Canada in Toronto at (416) 920-4916 for headache specialists in your area.

A list of headache specialists in the United Kingdom can be obtained by calling the Migraine Trust in London at 071-278 2676. In the United Kingdom, a letter of referral is needed from your doctor before an appointment can be made with a specialist.

In Australia, your doctor will have to refer you to a headache specialist. Many specialists are associated with the Australian headache clinics listed in Appendix III.

Before going to the doctor, write down a brief description of your headaches and how often you get them. Also include a history of medications you have taken or are taking. Office visits can be hurried and we sometimes forget important information.

If you do not get migraines very often the doctor may simply prescribe an anti-inflammatory medication, Midrin, codeine, sumatriptan, or some form of ergotamine. If your migraines are frequent, the doctor may start you on a daily dose of a beta blocker or an anti-inflammatory or antidepressant medication. If these medications do not work, a calcium channel blocker or Sansert may be prescribed. Outside of the United States, DHE nasal spray might be prescribed as an abortive agent, and, if daily preventative treatment is necessary, pizotifen might be recommended.

Treatment is usually a case of trial and error when it comes to migraine headaches. If your medication is not effective or you are having side effects, call your doctor. You have the right to be persistent until a medication that relieves your headaches can be found.

Most doctors will ask you to keep a monthly chart on which you will evaluate your migraine on a scale of 1 to 10 while on a particular medication. It is also a good idea to keep a record of your medications and their amounts so you won't repeat ineffective medications years later.

Keeping these kinds of records is part of taking charge of your own health. I have never had a doctor ask me about my diet, for example, even though the headache literature is full of warnings about amine-containing foods. Finding out about the interrelationship of diet, lifestyle, and migraine was up to me. I saw this information as part of becoming an informed consumer. Knowing your medication history is also part of becoming an informed consumer. Finding the right doctor is imperative, but he or she is only one part of your battle to overcome migraine. Total dependence on a doctor will only lead you down the garden path of continued misery.

You might tell a friend, lover, relative, or spouse you have decided to make a renewed effort to conquer your migraines. Ask this person to go to the doctor with you. Keep him or her informed about your medications and changes in your diet or lifestyle. Overcoming migraine is an adventure that can be tedious, and it is nice to have support along the way.

In summary, be patient, but relentless, in your search for a doctor who is knowledgeable and sympathetic. Migraine can be treated if you find the right doctor to work with you to achieve this goal.

10

Basic Steps in Treatment and Prevention

1. Become familiar with the medications used to treat migraine. Review Table 2.1 and the abortive drugs discussed in Appendix I.

2. If you get migraines more than once a week, you might need daily preventative medication. Review the drugs in Table 2.2 and the prophylactic medications discussed in Appendix I.

3. To get an overview of your medication history, make a list of all abortive and preventative medications you have taken. Note the dose and compare it to the dose recommended in Appendix I. Rank the effectiveness of each drug on a scale of 0 to 4, with 4 being the most effective. A drug would rate 0 if you had to stop its use because of side effects or because it wasn't effective. Make a separate list of the abortive and preventative migraine medications you have *not* taken. These lists will not only help you and your doctor better understand your medication history, they can also serve as a reference for future treatment plans.

4. You may have to stop eating amines, nitrites, MSG, sodium benzoate, and the sugar substitute aspartame. You might want to copy Table 3.1 and tape it to a cabinet door in the kitchen as a reminder.

5. Eliminate excessive or inconsistent use of coffee, tea, and caffeine to see if your headaches improve.

6. Do not go more than four hours without eating. Have a protein snack before going to bed.

7. Do not get too much or too little sleep.

8. To avoid withdrawal headaches, do not take more than 1000 mg of aspirin or acetaminophen daily and do not take ergotamine every day.

9. Avoid vitamin supplements for a month to see if headaches improve.

10. Have a complete physical examination to rule out headache as a symptom of an underlying disorder.

11. Stop taking birth control pills or estrogen replacement therapy to see if headaches improve.

12. You may want to keep a diary of all substances or conditions you experienced prior to a migraine attack. When a pattern emerges, you will know what triggers to avoid to prevent future attacks. The items in Tables 3.1 and 4.1 can be used as a guide when composing your diary.

13. Search until you find a knowledgeable and sensitive doctor who will be diligent in finding medication to abort and/or prevent your migraines.

14. If your medication is not working or has side effects, call your doctor. Be persistent until the right treatment for you can be found.

Migraine Portfolio

"Migraine Masterpieces" is the first art competition to be held in the United States on the subject of migraine. Each artist is a migraine sufferer. The work depicts the artist's conception of the debilitating effects of a migraine attack. The competition was sponsored by the National Headache Foundation and Wyeth-Ayerst Laboratories.

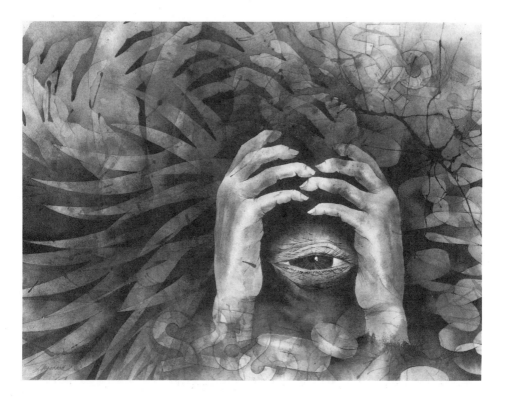

"Violent Passages" by Louise Woodard, Mattydale, NY. The artist focuses on the pain surrounding her eye and the confusion she has with numbers. First prize winner.

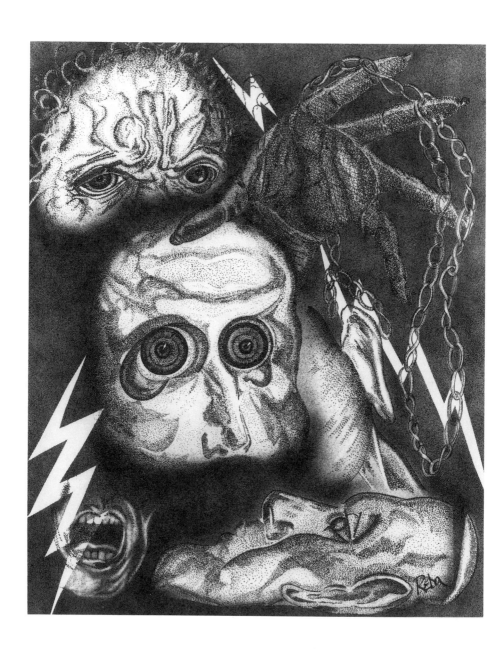

"Nemesis" by Rebecca Whitcanack, Moline, IL. The recurring phantom masks and chains represent the artist's fear of a migraine attack. The bolts of lightning symbolize the pain of migraine. Second prize winner.

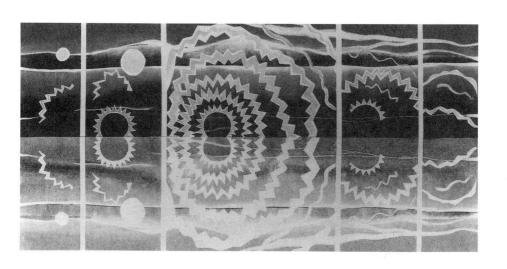

In "Reflections – Five Phases of a Shattered Scape" Carolyn Shaw, San Mateo, CA, portrays
the visual experiences of classical migraine.

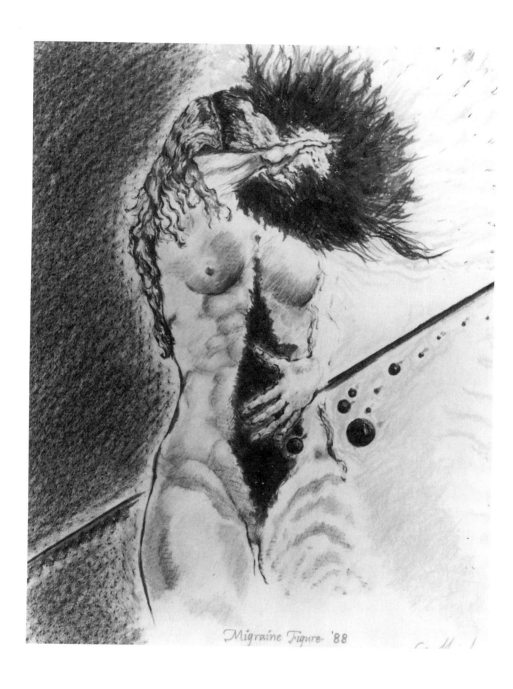

"Migraine Figure" by Constance Mariels, Davis, CA, depicts the exploding head pain and nausea of migraine. Third prize winner.

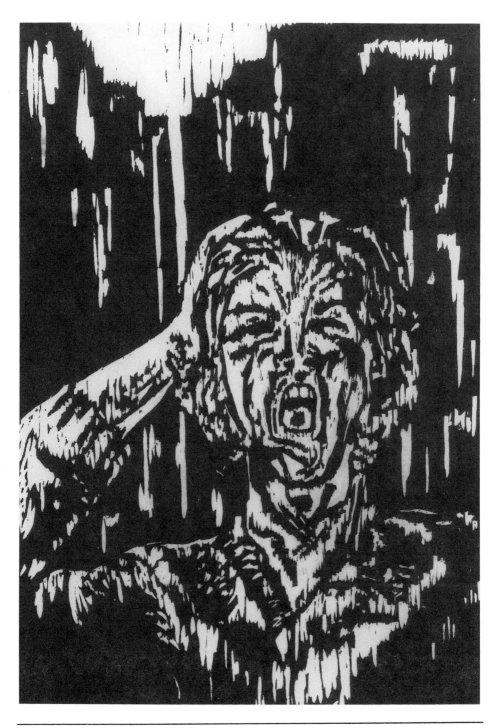

"Frustration, Self-Portrait" by Diane Wilkin, Morrisville, PA, captures the fear and frustration of a migraine attack.

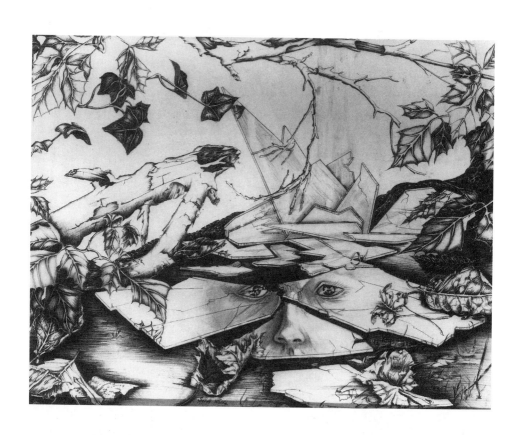

"Migraine" by Sarah Wolfe, Carmel, IN. According to the artist, "Even in the peace of the woods, distorting images, warping sounds —making you someone else — broken and on the ground."

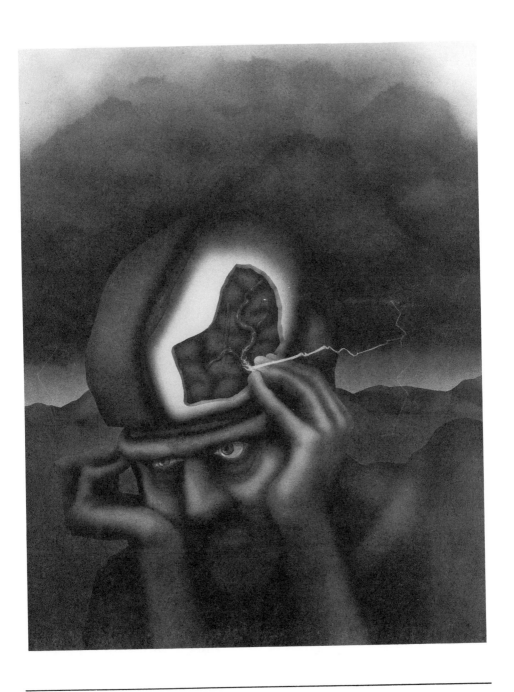

"The Storm Returns" by Thomas Wood, Salt Lake City, UT. In this work we can see how the artist's migraine attacks have depressed and eroded his well-being.

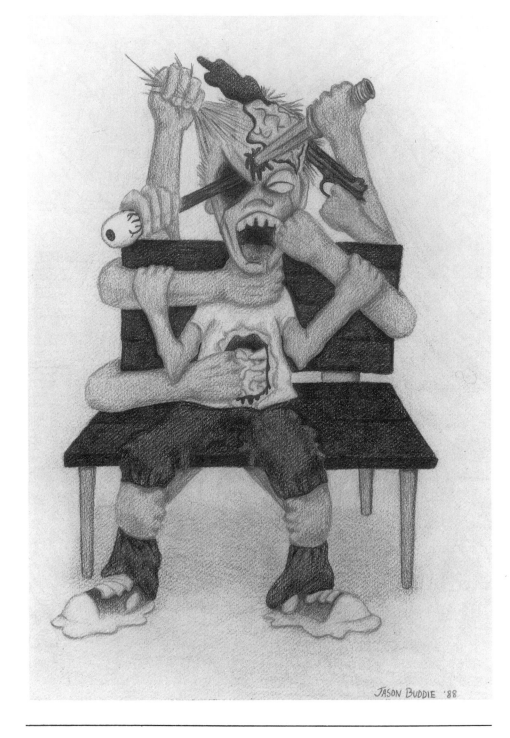

"A Migraine Headache" by Jason Buddie, Brunswick, OH. This young artist captures not only the explosive, wrenching, stabbing, nauseating effects of a migraine attack, but the sense of entrapment within the pain as well.

11

Children and Migraine

Migraine is the most common kind of headache in children. Symptoms may begin in infancy, with the average age of onset being 6 years. Forty percent of the children with migraine are female and 60 percent are male. By puberty these statistics change and migraine becomes more predominant in females. As these children reach adulthood, headaches may become less intense or may disappear altogether. In one study of children with migraine, 30 percent of the females and 52 percent of the males no longer had migraines by the age of 30.

Childhood migraine can have a variety of features. Such migraine symptoms as abdominal pain, nausea, vomiting, and vertigo may be more pronounced than the headache itself. The abdominal pain can be so severe it is mistaken for appendicitis. Many of these children have such sleep disturbances as nightmares, bed wetting, and sleep-walking. Almost half of the children with migraine also experience travel sickness. Convulsions are more common in young migraineurs than in adults with migraine. In atypical migraine, vomiting or abdominal pain may be unaccompanied by headache.

Migraine attacks may begin late in the day, in contrast to migraine in adults, which usually begins in the morning. Attacks occur less often and the length of the attack is shorter in children than in adults. Common migraine is more prevalent in children than classic migraine. Once children reach their teenage years their migraines become similar to those of the adult population.

Certain less common types of migraine may be accompanied by a number of neurological symptoms. Confusion, loss of balance, partial paralysis, numbness, tingling, lack of muscular coordination, speech abnormalities, and loss of consciousness are some of the symptoms that may be experienced by a minority of children. Visual disturbances may also accompany migraine and are especially predominant during the preheadache phase in classic migraine.

A variety of conditions can trigger a headache in children. Traveling, physical exercise, stress, a missed meal, and head injury are common headache triggers in the young migraineur. Additional triggers include noise, cold weather, and sudden changes in lighting such as going from a darkened room into the sunlight. The flickering light from television or movies can precipitate a headache. Increasing the lighting in the room while watching television is a good preventative measure.

Diet can be a migraine trigger for children as well as adults. Migraine can be precipitated in some children by the amine-containing foods that adults were cautioned to avoid in chapter 3.

It can be difficult to monitor a child's diet. In addition, the list of amine-containing foods is long, and children cannot be expected to have the discipline to avoid so many foods. Perhaps the best that can be hoped for is to eliminate those foods with the greatest headache provoking potential. Migraine sufferers were asked, in several studies, to list the foods that triggered their headaches. Cheese, chocolate, and citrus were rated as migraine precipitants by the most subjects. If children avoided at least these three foods, their headaches might be less severe. For example, many children begin each day with a glass of orange juice, a common headache trigger. Apple juice fortified with vitamin C could be served in its place, thus eliminating a daily migraine precipitant from the child's diet.

Children should be encouraged not to miss meals. Skipping lunch and eating a chocolate bar later in the day when hungry adds one trigger to another. This combination is likely to precipitate a headache in the food-sensitive migraineur. Even if headaches are not triggered by amine-containing foods, missing meals is a common cause of headaches in children.

Most neurologists do not believe migraine to be an allergic reaction to foods in the diet. They point out that children who improve on elimination diets, commonly given to counter allergies, do so because these diets often prohibit foods that contain vasoactive amines. Some allergists do not agree. They believe migraine can result from an immunologic reaction. According to these allergists, food may be reacted to as a foreign agent or antigen. Antibodies combine with the antigen to neutralize its toxic effect. The antigen-antibody reaction can result in skin rash, asthma, and rhinitis accompanied by paranasal pain.

Because allergy tests (skin prick and RAST) will not identify headache-provoking foods, the child is put on a diet of foods rarely known to produce an allergic reaction. Single foods are gradually added to the diet, and if no headache results, the food can be incorporated into the diet.

This diet, known as the oligoantigenic diet, is quite restrictive. It usually contains one or two sources of protein, one carbohydrate, one fruit, two or three vegetables, and a source of oil. Because growing children need variety in their diet, the oligoantigenic diet can be dangerous and must be monitored by a competent professional. Vitamin and mineral supplements will have to be taken. An anaphylactic reaction has been known to occur when an eliminated food was added back to the diet at a later date.

Foods to be used in an oligoantigenic diet can be found in Table 3.3 in chapter 3. Foods containing amines (Table 3.1), which I have seen listed in some oligoantigenic diets, should be avoided. One practitioner lists tofu on his oligoantigenic diet. Tofu is made from soy, a vasoactive amine that triggers headaches in food-sensitive migraineurs. If you take your child to an allergist, please select someone familiar with the role of vasoactive amines in migraine.

Children should not be subjected to the oligoantigenic diet unless they get migraines on a weekly basis. Improvement may take up to three weeks. As I said before, most neurologists are skeptical of these results. They believe some children may get migraines from amine-provoked vasodilation, but not from an antigen-antibody reaction. Only some foods contain amines, but to allergists all foods are possible antigens.

Headaches in children should not be ignored. The possible presence of serious illnesses that can cause headache must be investigated. Once these are ruled out and the headache is determined to be migraine, abortive or prophylactic treatment can begin.

Many children respond well to Tylenol (acetaminophen) as an abortive treatment for their headaches. Because of vomiting, analgesics in suppository form may be necessary. Aspirin should probably not be given to children because of its association with Reye's syndrome, a potentially fatal disease occurring in children under 15 years of age. According to some physicians, ergotamine should be avoided, especially in children under 6 years of age. Midrin (isometheptene mucate) has been used with success as an abortive agent in some children over 10 years of age.

Headaches in children who show seizure activity on an electroencephalogram (EEG) may be helped by such anticonvulsant medications as phenobarbital and Dilantin (phenytoin). A child can show seizure activity on an EEG and not actually have seizures. Some physicians feel that anticonvulsant medications have been helpful in eliminating migraines in children who do not have an abnormal EEG. Other physicians feel that anticonvulsants are contraindicated in nonepileptic children.

Periactin (cyproheptadine) is commonly used as a prophylactic treatment for childhood migraine. The side effects of Periactin include increased appetite, drowsiness, and dry mouth. This medication is contraindicated in children with asthma or a history of epilepsy. Inderal (propranolol) is another prophylactic medication that has been successful in preventing migraines in children. Some young migraineurs have also found pizotifen to be an effective preventive medication for migraine. The side effects of this drug include increased appetite and drowsiness. Pizotifen is not available in the United States. Because migraines can stop in children for no apparent reason, prophylactic medications are not usually administered beyond a six-month period. If spontaneous remission of the headache has occurred, treatment is no longer necessary.

Adolescents have been successfully treated with the antidepressant Elavil (amitriptyline). Clinical depression need not be a presenting symptom. Teenage girls may experience migraine for the first time when they begin to menstruate. Treatment for menstrual migraine is discussed in chapter 6. Adolescents can be treated with most of the medications used to treat migraine in adults.

Tigan (trimethobenzamide) and Compazine (prochlorperazine) have been used to relieve the nausea that may accompany migraine. The antinausea drug Reglan (metoclopramide) is usually contraindicated because it can cause sever extrapyramidal reactions in children. Extrapyramidal reactions include involuntary movements of the limbs and facial grimacing, as well as a host of other symptoms.

Children often respond well to nonpharmacological treatments. In one study using biofeedback, 28 out of 31 children found their migraines had improved. Headache frequency decreased by more than 70 percent. Sleep has been found to be a good abortive treatment for migraine. Many children who fall asleep during an attack find their migraine is gone when they awaken.

In summary, migraines are common in children, although the symptoms may differ from those experienced by adult migraineurs. Headaches in children should be taken seriously. Diseases that may be accompanied by headache should be ruled out before the headache is labeled as migraine. Sleep, medication, and biofeedback are effective methods of treating migraine in children. Preventative measures should be taken when possible. The young migraineur should be encouraged not to miss meals. Eliminating foods that trigger headaches may help prevent migraines in food-sensitive children.

12

Migraine and the Elderly

Migraines may continue into old age, may diminish in frequency and intensity, or may stop altogether. People can get migraines for the first time after the age of 60, but such experience is not common. The symptoms of migraine may change in the elderly. For example, people with classic migraine may continue to have the aura phase of their migraines, while the headache phase disappears as they advance in age. In another pattern, classic migraine may develop into common migraine. In this case, the aura phase is no longer experienced.

Headache can be a sign of a serious medical condition in the elderly. A complete physical examination is most important in this age group if headaches have just begun or if preexisting headaches change in intensity or characteristics. For example, what might be taken for a migraine equivalent in a younger person could well be the sign of an impending stroke in the older migraine sufferer.

Respiratory disease and high blood pressure are diseases of the elderly that may be accompanied by headache. In respiratory disease, increased carbon dioxide and decreased levels of oxygen in the blood can produce headaches. The blood vessels dilate in order to supply more oxygen to the brain. High blood pressure can cause headaches if the diastolic pressure exceeds 130 mmHg.

Giant cell arteritis and polymyalgia rheumatica may develop in people over 50 years of age. As noted in chapter 5, headache is one of the symptoms of these inflammatory diseases. Headache may also be one of the symptoms of renal disease, hypothyroidism, glaucoma, and anemia with hemoglobin below 10 g. Headaches may precede or follow a stroke.

Medications are a common cause of headaches in the elderly. Vasodilating drugs, such as nitroglycerin, and antiarrhythmics, such as digoxin, are used to treat heart disease. Headache is a well-known side effect of these medications. The headache-producing drugs reserpine and hydralazine are used to treat high blood pressure. Bronchodilators used in the treatment of respiratory disease and drugs used to treat Parkinson's disease may also trigger headaches.

Rheumatoid arthritis and degenerative spine disease may increase in severity as people age. These disorders are often treated with nonsteroidal anti-inflammatory drugs. Headache can be one of the side effects of these drugs.

I was given a variety of nonsteroidal anti-inflammatory medications during a flare-up of spinal stenosis in my lower back. Every drug I tried triggered a headache. Earlier I had taken Anaprox (naproxen) to treat my migraines. This anti-inflammatory drug also intensified my headaches. Low doses of aspirin seem to be the only anti-inflammatory I can tolerate. I even found ibuprofen in anti-inflammatory doses (over 1200 mg per day) to be a headache trigger.

Each of us reacts differently to these drugs. Some migraineurs might find the nonsteroidal anti-inflammatories to be helpful in treating headaches as well as in reducing the pain of rheumatoid arthritis or osteoarthritis. Do be aware, however, that these drugs can trigger or intensify headaches in some people.

Treating migraine in the elderly is more complicated than treatment in a younger population. The older people get, the more sensitive they become to the side effects of migraine medications. Dosages may have to be reduced to take this sensitivity into account. In addition, as health problems multiply in the elderly, migraine medications must be selected that do not exacerbate existing medical conditions.

Ergotamine is contraindicated in cases of high blood pressure, peripheral vascular disease, coronary heart disease, kidney or liver disease, and hyperthyroidism. In general, potent vasoconstricting drugs, such as ergotamine or Sansert (methysergide), are not usually used to treat headaches in the elderly because of the increased incidence of atherosclerotic disease in this age group. Tylenol (acetaminophen) cannot be used to abort headaches in people with renal or liver disease. Codeine will intensify the constipation often experienced by the elderly. Midrin (isometheptene mucate) has been suggested as a good abortive medication for migraine in the elderly. Midrin, however, is contraindicated if the migraineur has organic heart disease, glaucoma, peripheral vascular disease, severe kidney or liver disease, or high blood pressure.

Muscle relaxants have been used to abort the muscle contraction headache component of the mixed headache syndrome. Low doses of the muscle relaxant must be used because of the drug's tendency to cause sedation in the elderly.

The choice of a prophylactic migraine medication will also depend on coexisting health problems in the elderly migraineur. The beta blockers, especially Inderal (propranolol), are effective in the prophylactic treatment of migraine throughout the lifespan. Inderal and some of the other beta blockers can be given to migraineurs who also suffer from high blood pressure and heart disease. By using a drug that treats multiple disorders, the number of medications taken by the elderly can be reduced.

Calcium channel blockers, such as Isoptin (verapamil), have been successful in treating elderly migraineurs. Like the beta blockers, these drugs can serve a double purpose in that they are effective in the treatment of hypertension and some forms of heart disease as well as migraine.

The tricyclic antidepressants, such as Elavil (amitriptyline), Tofranil (imipramine), and Sinequan (doxepin), are used to treat both migraine and mixed headaches. Tricyclic antidepressants should not be used by people who suffer from cardiac arrhythmias or who have had a heart attack. The lowest possible dose of antidepressant medication should be used because of increased sensitivity to side effects in the elderly. For example, high doses of tricyclic antidepressants have been known to cause mental deterioration in elderly migraineurs. In addition, more time is needed for older people to become accustomed to dosage levels before these levels are raised.

In summary, a doctor should be consulted if headaches have just begun or if preexisting headaches change in intensity or characteristics. Medicines will have to be monitored. Headache can be a side effect of medications commonly taken by the elderly. Dosages of migraine medications may have to be reduced. Some migraine medications cannot be taken by people with disorders that may accompany the aging process. In general, increased vigilance is required as migraine sufferers advance in age.

13

Anecdotal Remedies

Anecdotal remedies helpful in the treatment of migraine gain popularity by word of mouth. Some are folk remedies that have been passed down from generation to generation. Other remedies are more recent. For the most part, extensive controlled experiments on the effectiveness of these remedies in migraine treatment have not been conducted. Many of the studies that have been undertaken involved a limited number of subjects and need to be repeated on a larger scale to verify their results. In many cases, we do not know how these remedies work or what their long-term safety might be.

People have been known to recommend a migraine treatment without thinking about the treatment's mode of action in the body. For example, niacin (nicotinic acid) is suggested as an abortive agent for migraine. Niacin is a vasodilator. If individuals with common migraine take niacin, their headaches will get worse. People with classic migraine, on the other hand, who take niacin during the aura phase, when vessels are constricted, may be able to abort a migraine attack.

Niacin is one of the B vitamins. Side effects may include a flushed face and itching skin. Migraineurs have taken 50 mg at the first sign of an aura, followed by another 50 mg if the aura is not aborted. Taking more than 100 mg of niacin at any one time may cause a toxic reaction. Niacin is contraindicated in cases of severe diabetes, liver disease, ulcers, or glaucoma. It should not be combined with Catapres (clonidine).

Caffeine has the opposite effect of niacin. Caffeine is a vasoconstrictor. Taken during the aura phase of classic migraine, caffeine would not be helpful; but if it is taken during the headache phase of classic or common migraine, when the vessels are dilated, it can be an effective abortive agent. In other words, the aim is to enlarge constricted vessels during the aura phase by taking a vasodilator and to reduce dilated vessels during the headache phase by taking a vasoconstrictor. To avoid a rebound headache, do not take more than 200 mg of caffeine daily or, if more is consumed, do not let 12 hours go by without some caffeine intake.

Drinking black coffee is a common folk remedy for migraine. Because of its amine content, coffee should be avoided by food- sensitive migraineurs. It is the caffeine in the coffee that helps the headache. People trying to avoid amine-containing foods or drinks can take one or, at the most, two 100 mg caffeine tablets as an abortive measure.

Magnesium has been found to help some headache sufferers. This mineral can act as a calcium channel blocker. By preventing the entry of calcium into the cells, magnesium may block vasoconstriction. Low magnesium levels have been found during migraine attacks. A calcium channel blocker is a vasodilator and may intensify a migraine if it is taken once the headache is underway. The same may be true of magnesium.

How effective is magnesium in the treatment of migraine? In a study at East Tennessee State University, a majority of subjects who took 200 mg of magnesium found their migraines had improved. Three hundred of the women in the study were pregnant. Another 60 subjects were taking oral contraceptives. Magnesium is known to be particularly low in these special groups. A more representative cross section of migraineurs needs to be tested to verify magnesium's effectiveness in migraine treatment.

Magnesium is available in many forms, including magnesium gluconate and magnesium oxide tablets. Magnesium should not be taken in chelated form. Chelated minerals have been combined with amino acids, and these amino acids may produce headaches in amine-sensitive individuals.

The fish oil known as omega-3 is reputed to decrease the intensity of migraine headaches. Omega-3 reduces platelet serotonin release and is believed to have anti-inflammatory properties. In a study at the University of Cincinnati Medical Center, omega-3 reduced migraine intensity, but it did not appear to entirely eliminate migraines. Two of 8 female subjects in the study had a reduction in headache intensity greater than 33 percent. Five of the 7 male subjects experienced a reduction in headache intensity greater than 33 percent. Four of the subjects taking omega-3 found that their migraines had become worse. This study was small and needs to be repeated on a larger scale before conclusions can be drawn about the effectiveness of omega-3 in migraine treatment.

The dose used in the above study was 15 g of MaxEPA per day. The manufacturer, on the other hand, suggests that only 6 g be taken per day (two MaxEPA capsules three times per day). Each MaxEPA capsule contains 1000 mg, or 1 g, of fish oil. One MaxEPA capsule contains 5 mg of cholesterol. Promega and Proto-Chol are other sources of omega-3 that are essentially cholesterol-free. The omega-3 fatty acids are known as EPA and DHA. One capsule of Promega or Proto-Chol contains more EPA and the same amount of DHA as one capsule of MaxEPA. Because of the high dosage suggested, cod liver oil and other fish oil products containing large amounts of vitamin A or vitamin D should be avoided.

The aura associated with classic migraine can be stopped, in some cases, by breathing into a paper bag. In a study by S.L. Dexter, reported in the *British Medical Journal*, 5 out of 8 migraine attacks were aborted by rebreathing carbon dioxide. Dexter's study was based on the theory that hyperventilation plays a role in migraine development. One can speculate, however, that rebreathing carbon dioxide and decreasing oxygen intake may induce vasodilation, thus reversing the vasoconstriction that causes the preheadache symptoms of classic migraine. The subjects in Dexter's study practiced rebreathing from 15 to 20 minutes before their symptoms were aborted. In a later study by A. Pradalier and his associates, 29 out of 113 migraines were aborted by rebreathing carbon dioxide during the aura phase of the attack.

As noted in chapter 2, feverfew has been widely used in England in the prevention of migraine. Beginning as a folk remedy, it has continued to gain in popularity as a migraine treatment. Research on the effectiveness of feverfew has increased over the last several years.

In one survey of feverfew users, 70 percent said they experienced improvement while taking the herb. Migraines were completely eliminated in 33 percent of those surveyed. In a 1988 study of feverfew at University Hospital in Nottingham, 24 percent of 59 subjects found their migraines had decreased in frequency and intensity, but the length of the attack had not changed. Migraine was not totally eliminated in any of the subjects in the second study.

No one is quite sure how feverfew helps to prevent migraines. Prostaglandins seem to be implicated in this process. Prostaglandins are a group of compounds synthesized in the body from fatty acids. These compounds play a role in causing inflammation. Feverfew inhibits the synthesis of prostaglandins. Researchers speculate it is feverfew's anti-inflammatory action that makes it an effective migraine treatment for some people. Feverfew's capacity to inhibit platelet serotonin release may also be related to its ability to prevent migraines. More research will have to be done before feverfew's role in migraine prevention is fully comprehended. The safety of feverfew for long-term use is not known.

The suggested dose by one manufacturer is one or two 125 mg capsules of freeze-dried feverfew daily. Side effects, experienced by a small number of people taking the fresh herb, include mouth ulcers, itchy skin, and a sore throat. Side effects from the freeze-dried form are rare.

Edema, or fluid retention, may accompany a migraine attack. Urinating a copious amount of fluid can signal the end of the attack. Is the edema the cause of the migraine? Most authorities think not, because a diuretic that eliminates edema does not help prevent migraines. Eliminating salt in the diet should have the same effect as the diuretic: it would reduce the edema, but it would not prevent migraines. It is curious, therefore, that one researcher found migraine improvement to be directly linked to salt intake.

In a study by J.B. Brainard, reported in *Headache Quarterly*, 85 migraine subjects were placed on a low salt diet. None of the subjects were taking prophylactic medications. Ninety-four percent found their migraines had improved on the low salt diet. It should be noted that Brainard's subjects were restricted to a diet that eliminated tyramine, MSG, and nitrites, as well as reducing the amount of salt. We cannot be sure it was the salt alone that produced the decrease in headache frequency and intensity. Brainard had established the connection between migraine and salt in an earlier study in which he found he could induce headaches in his subjects by giving them capsules containing 1 g of salt.

Salt is not mentioned in the literature as a migraine trigger. As stated earlier, most clinicians assume that because diuretics do not help migraine, lowering salt levels will also do little to decrease migraine attacks. Brainard's work would lead us to believe that previous assumptions about the role of salt as a migraine precipitant may have to be reevaluated.

The anecdotal remedies discussed in this chapter and their treatment goals are outlined in Table 13.1

Table 13.1
Anecdotal Remedies

REMEDY	TREATMENT GOAL
Niacin	Aborts aura phase in classic migraine
Caffeine	Aborts headache in classic and common migraine
Magnesium	Migraine prophylactic
Omega-3	Prophylactic treatment. May reduce severity of migraine
Breathing into a paper bag	Aborts aura phase in classic migraine
Feverfew	Migraine prophylactic
Salt reduction	Migraine prophylactic

In summary, the remedies discussed in this chapter have been of some help in relieving migraines. Although most of these remedies have been beneficial in only a minority of cases, you could be one of the fortunate migraine sufferers who will be helped. They may be worth trying, especially if you have had trouble with the more traditional medications. It is unclear whether combining these remedies with other medications would reduce their effectiveness, or if such a combination would be safe. You should check with your doctor before trying any of these treatments. Medical conditions might exist that would prohibit their use.

14

Unorthodox Treatments

Homeopathy and Oriental medicine have helped some migraine sufferers. These approaches to disease are unorthodox, not because they are ineffective, but because they are not part of mainstream medicine in Western society.

Homeopathic medicine was developed by the German physician Samuel Hahnemann in the nineteenth century. According to Hahnemann, symptoms are an indication the body is trying to rid itself of disease. By encouraging these symptoms, rather than suppressing them, Hahnemann believed patients would become well. For example, after eating spoiled food you might experience nausea and a desire to vomit. A homeopathic practitioner would view the vomiting as an effort by the body to rid itself of the toxic substance. A Western physician, on the other hand, would prescribe medication to stop the nausea and vomiting. Traditional doctors view disease as a combination of symptoms that are to be reversed. Homeopathic practitioners view symptoms as the body's method of healing itself.

After taking quinine, Hahnemann developed the symptoms of malaria. From this simple experiment he formulated the Law of Similars. According to this law, a remedy can cure a disease if it produces the symptoms of the disease in a healthy person. Hippocrates illustrated this principle when he said, "Through the like, disease is produced and through the application of the like, it is cured." By giving various animal, vegetable, and mineral substances to healthy people, Hahnemann was able to discover which symptoms were associated with a particular substance. This substance could then be used to cure a sick person with the same symptoms.

Homeopathic practitioners look at the total person when prescribing treatments. The patient's general physical condition, mental and emotional characteristics, life style, medical history, and specific symptoms are taken into consideration. Migraine treatment will differ, depending on the individual characteristics and medical history of the patient.

Homeopathic treatments are available in a variety of greatly diluted solutions. The number of times they are vigorously shaken, or "succcessed," also varies. The number and letter following the name of the medicine indicates its dilution and succession. Bryonia 30X tells us the original tincture of bryonia was diluted 30 times, with one part of every new solution being mixed with nine parts of distilled water or alcohol. Bryonia would be successed before each of the 30 dilutions. Hahnemann felt that these greatly diluted solutions eliminated side effects while retaining the remedy's therapeutic properties. After so much dilution only the energy field of the original substance remains. Homeopaths believe cure takes place when the energy field of a remedy matches the energy field of the ill person. Like resonating with like generates the energy needed to overcome illness and restore harmony.

Treating acute conditions is a relatively simple matter. Treating chronic conditions is much more complicated. Hahnemann believed chronic illness can be influenced by unresolved childhood diseases as well as diseases inherited from one's ancestors. If childhood diseases were treated with harsh medicines that only eliminated symptoms, the disease itself might never have been resolved and would continue to influence a person's health. Inherited weaknesses, which Hahnemann called "miasms," can also continue to influence the present-day health of the patient. In order to treat chronic illness, the practitioner prescribes constitutional remedies that remove these remnants from the past.

The Law of Cure is another important concept in homeopathy. According to this law, symptoms move from vital organs to those that are less vital and from organs deep in the body to those nearer the surface. The Law of Cure also states that symptoms disappear in the reverse order of their chronological appearance. For example, the patient might have had hay fever as a child. The hay fever disappeared in adulthood, only to be replaced by migraines. While being treated for migraines, the patient may temporarily develop the symptoms of hay fever. Current symptoms may get worse before improving. If this happens, it can be assumed the remedy has been effective and treatment can be discontinued. Symptoms should disappear in short order. The brief return of past illness and the temporary worsening of present symptoms are part of the natural progression toward health.

A homeopathic remedy must be taken between meals. If the medicine is in pill form, a single pill should be poured into the cap of the bottle and inserted into the mouth from the cap. The pill should not be touched with the hands, but allowed to dissolve in the mouth without being washed down with water or other liquids. All foods, liquids, toothpaste, and smoking should be avoided for at least 20 minutes after taking a homeopathic remedy. It is suggested that coffee, tea, alcohol, and substances containing camphor (Chap Stick, for example) should be avoided altogether. Some practitioners want the patient to stop using other medicines while taking a homeopathic remedy.[1] Other practitioners permit their use as long as the medicine is taken at least 20 minutes after the homeopathic remedy. Substances used in homeopathic treatment are very sensitive and can be easily rendered inactive if these suggestions are not followed.

A selection of homeopathic remedies and the kinds of headaches they are used to treat is presented in Table 14.1. Out of the more than 2000 homeopathic remedies, several may treat similar headaches. The one that is right for you will depend on your medical history and individual characteristics, as well as your headache symptoms.

Finding the right practitioner is very important. If possible, try to find a practitioner who has graduated from a four-year school of homeopathy. Medical doctors who have taken a short course in homeopathy are licensed to practice homeopathy in some countries. These doctors will know more about traditional medical science, but less about homeopathy, than a nonmedical practitioner who has studied for four years at a homeopathic school.

---

1. Do not stop taking any medicine before consulting with your doctor. Such a practice could be very dangerous.

Table 14.1

Homeopathic Headache Remedies

REMEDY	HEADACHE SYMPTOMS
Belladonna	Throbbing headache accompanied by a red, flushed face. Scalp is sensitive to the touch
Bryonia	A right-sided headache that is bursting or throbbing in nature. Movement, such as bending over, intensifies the headache
Gelsemium	Headache feels like a band around the head. Pain extends into the neck
Iris versicolor	Begins with a blurring of vision and develops into a migraine-like headache
Kali bichromicum	A sinus-like headache with pain a around the eyes
Nux vomica	A hangover headache
Sanguinaria canadensis	Headache over right eye accompanied by nausea, vomiting, and dizziness

A list of homeopathic practitioners in the United States, United Kingdom, Canada, Australia, and New Zealand can be obtained by contacting the following organizations. In the United Kingdom, homeopathic medical doctors and nonmedical registered practitioners are represented by separate organizations.

United States
International Foundation
for Homeopathy
2366 East Lake Avenue
East 301
Seattle, WA 98102
Telephone: (206) 324-8230

United Kingdom

The Faculty of Homoeopathy
The Royal London
Homoeopathic Hospital
Great Ormond Street
London WC1N 3HR
Telephone: (01) 837 3091
(Homeopathic medical doctors)

The Society of Homoeopaths
2 Artizan Road
Northampton   NN1 4HU
Telephone: 604 21400
(Nonmedical registered
practitioners)

Canada
International Society for
the Promotion of Homeopathy
2246 Spruce Street
Vancouver
British Columbia V6H2P3
Telephone: (604) 732-7276

Australia
Australian Federation of
Homeopaths
21 Bulah Close
Berowra Heights
New South Wales 2082
Telephone: (2) 456-3602

New Zealand
Homeopathic Society, Inc.
P.O. Box 67/095
Mt. Eden
Auckland 1031

Chinese medicine is viewed as an unorthodox treatment modality in the West, although it has been used for centuries to treat disease in China. No brief discussion can adequately describe Chinese medicine. It would take volumes to illustrate in any depth the nearly 5000-year history of traditional medicine in China. Nevertheless, some information on the background of this approach will be presented to aid your evaluation of Chinese medicine as a possible treatment for migraine.

The concept of Qi (pronounced "chee") and the principle of Yin/Yang are basic to an understanding of traditional Chinese medicine. Qi is the energy, or life force, in the human body. Qi flows through channels in the body called meridians. It controls the functioning of the individual's physical, mental, emotional, and spiritual processes. Too much or too little Qi results in ill health. In a healthy person, the proper amount of Qi is flowing unimpeded. When Qi becomes blocked, or misdirected, disease results.

Yin and Yang represent contrasting forces that are interdependent. Together they form a whole. One cannot exist without the other. Day is Yang, night is Yin. Cold is Yin, hot is Yang. Female is Yin and male is Yang. Yet each female also contains Yang and each male also contains Yin. The solid organs in the body are Yin and the hollow organs are Yang. The channels carrying Qi unite all of the Yin/Yang organs. When Yin and Yang are not in balance, Qi does not flow smoothly. Pairs of organs and their Yin/Yang classification are presented in Table 14.2

The one concept uniting the principles of Chinese medicine is balance. To maintain good health, there cannot be too much or too little Qi. Yin and Yang must be in harmony. Diagnosis in traditional Chinese medicine is a process of detecting imbalance.

Two important diagnostic procedures performed by a practitioner trained in traditional Chinese medicine are an examination of the patient's tongue and an analysis of his or her pulses. The tongue reflects the state of one's health. Imbalances within the body can be determined by the appearance of the tongue. The practitioner will also feel for six pulses in each of the patient's wrists. These pulses correspond to the internal organs. In addition, the practitioner will note the patient's appearance, complexion, respiratory sounds and body odor. The practitioner will ask questions about thirst, sensitivity to heat and cold, appetite, perspiration, fever, sleep patterns, and food likes and dislikes. Appearance, sound, smell, the answers to the above questions, and an examination of the tongue and pulses will enable the practitioner to determine which underlying imbalance is producing the patient's symptoms. A person with migraine, for example, might be diagnosed as having an excessive liver Yang (the liver being a Yin organ). A liver with too much Yang will produce a stagnation of Qi. After a certain amount of accumulation, Qi explodes upwards, creating pressure and pain in the head. Treatment would be directed toward reducing the Yang of the liver.

Acupuncture, acupressure massage, and herbal remedies are three of several treatment modalities used in traditional Chinese medicine. All treatment is directed toward restoring balance by manipulating the flow of Qi. In acupuncture, very fine needle are inserted into points on the channels carrying Qi. Through this procedure, the practitioner can unblock or redirect the flow of Qi.

Acupressure massage (called shiatsu in Japan) is used most often in Chinese clinics to treat patients complaining of back pain or tension headaches. In this form of treatment, pressure is applied to trigger points on the skin. Acupressure massage gives temporary relief. It does not appear to have the more lasting effects of acupuncture or herbal remedies.

Table 14.2

Yin/Yang Organ Pairs

ORGAN PAIRS	YIN/YANG
Heart	Yin
Small intestine	Yang
Spleen	Yin
Stomach	Yang
Lungs	Yin
Colon	Yang
Kidney	Yin
Bladder	Yang
Liver	Yin
Gall bladder	Yang

Herbal medicines are a common treatment for migraines in China. Remedies may contain as many as 12 herbs.[1] These ingredients work together to correct the imbalance that is at the root of the headache. Many patients prefer herbal remedies to Western medicine because of the absence of side effects. Because no two patients are alike, prescriptions will differ for each migraine sufferer.

A practitioner who uses acupuncture or herbal remedies to correct imbalance in the body becomes proficient after years of study. Using acupuncture as a method of pain control requires less training. Pain control is in the Western tradition of giving symptom relief. Treating the root cause of the problem is the goal of traditional Chinese medicine and, according to most practitioners, results in a more effective cure than simply treating the symptom. According to these practitioners, just treating a symptom, such as pain, without looking at the entire system could do injury to the organs from which energy was removed in order to overcome the pain.

As we saw in chapter 8, much of the acupuncture used to treat migraine in the West has not been very successful. When acupuncture is used by Western physicians to eliminate pain, the placement of the needles is often according to a set formula that does not differ from patient to patient. The diagnostic procedures used by practitioners trained in traditional Chinese medicine are based on individual characteristics that do not lend themselves to acupuncture by formula. A physician who has taken a short course in acupuncture has to practice by formula. He or she cannot possibly have the knowledge it has taken a practitioner trained in traditional methods years to perfect. Acupuncture can help migraine sufferers if the practitioner has the proper training and is not offering pain control based on the placement of needles according to a formula. Formula acupuncture does not recognize individual differences, nor does it take into consideration the root cause of the problem.

In the United States, many states require the passing of a state licensing examination before a person can practice acupuncture in that state. By passing a national licensing examination an acupuncturist can receive additional certification. Please make sure your acupuncturist is certified on either the state or national level. In some states, medical doctors who have taken a short course in acupunture,

---

1. Herbal remedies containing licorice or ginseng should be avoided by amine-sensitive migraineurs.

as opposed to the usual three-year program, do not have to be certified. These doctors practice formula acupuncture and have not had much long-term success in the treatment of migraine. Practitioners who have had at least three years of training and have been certified on the national level are registered with the National Commission for the Certification of Acupuncturists. Practitioners who have been authorized by state law or national examination to practice acupuncture belong to the American Association of Acupuncture and Oriental Medicine.

Some acupuncture schools in the West teach herbal medicine as well as acupuncture. If you would like a practitioner with a more eclectic approach, ask the practitioner if he or she has been trained in herbal medicine and offers this modality in addition to acupuncture.

A list of qualified practitioners in the United States, Canada, the United Kingdom, Australia, and New Zealand can be obtained by contacting the following organizations.

United States

National Commission for the
Certification of Acupuncturists
1424 16 Street NW
Suite 105
Washington, DC 20036
Telephone: (202) 232-1404

American Association of
Acupuncture and Oriental
Medicine
1424 16 Street NW, Suite 105
Washington, DC 20036
Telephone: (202) 265-2287

Canada

Acupuncture Foundation
of Canada
5 Roughfield Crescent
Toronto
Ontario M1S4K3
Telephone: (416) 291-4317

United Kingdom

British Acupuncture
Association
8 Hunter Street
London WC1N 1BN
Telephone: 071-833 8164

The Traditional Acupuncture
Society
11 Grange Park
Strafford-Upon-Avon
Warwickshire
Telephone: 0789 298798

Australia

Australian Acupuncture
Association
P.O. Box 1744
Brisbane
Queensland 4001
Telephone: (7) 221-6960

New Zealand

New Zealand Registrar
of Acupuncturists, Inc.
Birkenhead Health Centre
235 Onewa Road
Birkenhead
Auckland
Telephone: 4802255

Registrar
Hamilton Acupuncture Clinic
113 Aberdeen Drive
Hamilton
Telephone: 73013

In summary, the medical approaches in this chapter offer certain advantages over Western medicine as it is commonly practiced. Symptoms are not treated as an end in themselves, but are viewed within the context of the whole person. The remedies used by homeopathic practitioners and the herbs and other treatments used by traditional Chinese practitioners are nontoxic. Unlike Western medicines, they have no side effects.

I have had no direct experience with either homeopathy or traditional Chinese medicine. Studies on the use of traditional Chinese medicine in migraine treatment are meager and contradictory. Only one study using homeopathic medicines in migraine treatment has been conducted. The 60 patients in the study experienced a "significant reduction" in the frequency and intensity of their headaches. The scarcity of scientific data is countered by the enthusiastic testimony of practitioners on the effectiveness of their respective methods in migraine treatment. Such testimony merits investigation.

15

Sharing Information

I would like to thank the following readers for sharing their experiences. Their letters have greatly enriched the second edition of this book.

Dear Betsy:

I am 52 years old. I have been having migraines since 1964. They have changed in that they have become more frequent, more severe, and longer lasting. My headaches are so bad, I am unable to function in my capacity as an LPN here in Florida.

The length of the headache depends on what time of day I get the symptoms. If I get the headache during my waking hours, I can take part of a Cafergot suppository which will prevent the symptoms from becoming full-blown. If I get a headache during the night the pain usually awakens me and I am not aware of how long I have had the headache. By taking Cafergot upon awakening I can sometimes get rid of the pain within 2 hours or (and this is the worst part) it can last for as long as 24 hours, and in some instances, for 48 hours.

The pain is difficult to describe. I know I cannot lift my head from the pillow. I do not want any noise around or any upsets. Generally, I just want to be left alone. There are times when a vibrator will diminish the pain but it returns when I stop the treatment. Ice packs on my neck and the top of my head are also helpful. I do not have any visual problems but I do have nausea which can be persistent.

Over the years I have seen neurologists, internists, an acupuncturist, holistic practitioners, and chiropractors. Medications I have taken include Ergostat, Fiorinal, Inderal, Isoptin, Procardia, Elavil, Midrin, Phenergan, and Cafergot. Only Cafergot suppositories have helped me. Biofeedback and acupuncture were not effective. I have had a series of brain scans and all sorts of medical tests in an attempt to discover what was the cause of my problem. All were negative. Every doctor I consulted attributed my headaches to stress. However, I did not have any stress in my life at the time which made this explanation untenable.

Recently, I began to notice I was becoming ill after eating certain foods. I went to a Wellness Center where a sample of my blood was taken for examination by an immunology laboratory. The results showed I had a food sensitivity to bananas, kidney beans, eggs, green beans, mushrooms, lamb, lobster, and yellow beans. None of these was sufficiently high on the Immuno 1 Blood Print for the treating physician to believe that they would cause migraines, but they did show a reactive reading and it was suggested that I avoid them.

Vivonex was given to me by a food allergist to take prior to inducing foods into my system that might be suspect for allergies. Why do you think I had three migraines the week I was on this nutritional diet? I feel certain my migraines are related to my diet, especially foods containing Yellow Dye Number 5, preservatives, and artificial flavors. I do not understand why I would have migraines when taking Vivonex since it is supposed to be a pure nutrient. I would be most grateful if you could offer any insight into this dilemma.

Susanne Page
Sarasota, Florida

Dear Susanne:

You seem to be on the right track in equating migraine with your diet. The foods that cause migraine are not necessarily the foods we are allergic to. In an allergic reaction, antibodies are formed causing such symptoms as rashes and asthma. Migraine comes from food containing substances that some people cannot metabolize. You probably got migraines from Vivonex because it contains vasoactive amines. Allergists are not always helpful when it comes to migraine. They have been known to put us on diets containing migraine-producing amines. Our problems do not stem from allergy, they come from the inability to metabolize certain amines, nitrites, aspartame, MSG, and some food preservatives and colorings. We do not produce antibodies to these substances as in a true allergic reaction. Instead, toxic levels build up causing the blood vessels in the brain to dilate. Such dilation causes the symptoms of migraine. (See chapter 11 for a discussion of allergy and migraine.)

Dear Betsy:

This letter is an update on the status of my migraines. I hope you will find what I offer useful, but even more important, I hope you will respond with any information you may have regarding questions that have arisen since I last wrote to you.

By avoiding some of the foods that you have listed—specifically, freshly squeezed orange juice or orange slices, freshly baked yeast breads and rolls, pumpkin and sunflower seeds, aged cheeses, sour cream, sodium benzoate, and MSG—I had greatly diminished the occurrence of my headaches. However, this fall I went through quite a siege of headache symptoms which were always controlled if I took Cafergot in time. The only time I really got a bad headache was at night if I did not wake up in time to take the suppository. (I only need a third of a Cafergot suppository to avoid a headache.)

A friend and I went on a cruise and in order to survive eating foods with contents unknown, and as a preventive, I took a piece of Cafergot every night. No headaches.

Recently I was encouraged to go to an internist who was supposedly an excellent diagnostician. The internist was very upset with the amount of ergotamine I was taking, even though I had been told that 10 mg (or five suppositories) a week was O.K. She told me to stop all treatment and she put me on the following medications:

1. Anaprox—274 mg three times daily,
2. Elavil—10 mg at bedtime.

I followed this treatment for 8 days without a headache, but on the ninth day I was working outside pruning (overexerting myself which 3 years ago always produced a headache) and I got very ill. Just before the migraine came on I was feeling nauseous and completely debilitated. The next day, after taking Darvocet plus 25 mg of Xanax for the headache with no relief, I got the same debilitated feeling and took Cafergot. The Cafergot got me through without a headache, so I stopped the new medication cold.

The internist's comments about Cafergot frightened me so I called a druggist whom I know who said, "If you can stop a migraine with no more than two and one-half suppositories a week I cannot see the danger." The internist said I could develop nerve damage or hypertension. She said the prolonged use of ergotamine was very dangerous. Do you have any information on Cafergot dosages? Don't you agree that if so little works for me I should watch my diet and use it when necessary?

I am almost convinced that food is a trigger for my migraines. If I am careful—and how difficult that is when one eats out a great deal—about what I eat and how much and how often I consume the foods that you have listed as triggering migraines, I can minimize the number of headaches I have. Do you have any information as to where I can be tested for these food sensitivities so that I can more narrowly define what they are? Right now some of it is hit or miss. For example, we purchased a bread machine and I started baking homemade breads and rolls and was getting a mid-day headache. It took a month to discover it was the yeast that I was using in the baked goods that triggered the headache. In another case, I purchased a pure cereal (Granola). After eating it for breakfast, I got a migraine. The cereal contains two seeds on your list, so I gave it up.

One last thing regarding my diet. When I started to get the headaches last fall, I had given up my two cups of caffeine a day and had started drinking decaf. By going back on caffeine I have reduced my daily migraine symptoms.

Susanne Page
Sarasota, Florida

Dear Susanne:

What your new internist seems to be doing is to have you stop using abortive medicine (ergotamine) as a preventative treatment for migraine. She has replaced Cafergot with two common preventative medications (Anaprox and Elavil). If you can tolerate these two drugs they are worth trying for a couple of months to see if your migraines are reduced (reduction may be the goal, not stopping migraines altogether). It doesn't seem you gave Elavil and Anaprox a fair trial.

To prevent rebound headaches, do not take Cafergot two days in a row. According to one headache authority, migraine sufferers should not take more than 10 mg of Cafergot per week. Bellergal-S, on the other hand, contains such a small amount of ergotamine (0.6 mg), it can be taken daily. The reaction to ergotamine can be unpredictable. Chronic rebound headaches have developed in some patients using as little as 0.5 mg daily. Because a variety of medical disorders preclude the use of ergotamine, you should not be taking even a small dose on a daily basis without a physician's supervision. Ergotamine can have dangerous side effects and should be used only as prescribed. Patients taking ergotamine need to be monitored for signs of toxicity. Your questions about ergotamine are good ones, but they need to be discussed with a physician specializing in migraine treatment who can oversee your use of this drug.

No one can test you for foods that trigger migraines. Tests only show antibody reactions and these foods do not produce antibodies. They produce vasodilation and no test for this exists. Symptoms are the only indication that vasodilation is present. If you have noticed that some of the foods on my list trigger a migraine, you can assume all of these foods are suspect.

Be careful of caffeine. To avoid a rebound headache, either keep your intake to under 200 mg or do not let more than 12 hours go by without some caffeine. Caffeine is a mild vasoconstrictor.

You mentioned your relapse was caused by exertion. This didn't make sense until I realized your pruning was done under the hot Florida sun. The sun beating down on my head will trigger a terrible migraine unless I wear a hat and sunglasses. The next time you work outdoors, try wearing a hat. I suspect it was the sun and not exertion that caused your relapse.

You might want to go to one of the headache centers listed in Appendix III. As an alternative you might think about calling the National Headache Foundation (1-800-843-2256) for a list of doctors in your area who belong to the foundation. In my opinion, because of the frequency of your attacks, you should consider seeing a physician specializing in migraine treatment.

Dear Betsy:

From ages 5 to 20, my major migraine symptom was nausea, usually without vomiting; I'd also get very pale and dizzy and would feel hot or cold; I saw "spots" but seldom had head pain. These episodes occurred about once a month and lasted approximately 4 hours. As I got older, they became more frequent, lasted longer, and gradually included headache.

By early adulthood the attacks occurred several times a week, lasted about a day, and involved more head pain than nausea. Visual disturbances became rare, and my moods rose and fell suddenly, in synch with the rhythms of an episode.

At the age of 46, my migraines are chronic but manageable. When I avoid all triggers, migraine is experienced as dull, temporary neck and head pain that often can be aborted through medication, stretching and relaxation exercises, hot baths, and ice packs. If I cannot abort the attack, the main symptom is head pain (4 to 8 hours); nausea is extremely rare.

Over the years, a variety of migraine triggers have come to my attention. Monosodium glutamate and sodium nitrite have triggered attacks all my life. More recently, I have found aspartame to be a migraine trigger. I avoid these three substances like the plague and read all packaging carefully (even the aspartame in breath mints has laid me low). "Natural flavoring" is often another way to say MSG and so is "hydrolyzed vegetable protein." Alcohol continues to be a certain trigger.

Weather conditions—especially quick changes in humidity or barometric pressure—often cause attacks. I use more medication in roughly February to March and August to September, when weather conditions are changing into a less stable pattern.

However one labels it, stress (tension, emotions) plays a role and sometimes seems to be the sole trigger. In particular, anger and pressures of time are a problem, but I can't say which comes first: Am I angry/pressured because of migraine, or do I have migraine because of anger/pressure? And what about the majority of the attacks, in which emotions seem inconsequential? This area is a conundrum.

Treatment has progressed in tandem with my changing migraine patterns. As a child I was tested for allergies, but nothing specific or helpful emerged. I combated nausea by lying still in a dark, warm place. As head pain evolved, I added aspirin and its over-the-counter equivalents; none of these ever alleviated the pain.

As a young adult I added induced vomiting to my arsenal by drinking a large glass of very warm saltwater; I'd feel better for a while after vomiting, perhaps well enough to fall asleep. Then I discovered that an ice cube helped ease the specific locus of pain, and that immersing myself in a hot bath drew blood to my extremities and helped me relax.

When I finally consulted a doctor, I learned that the problem was indeed migraine and that by avoiding trigger foods and alcohol, and using Cafergot suppositories, my symptoms could be reduced. The Cafergot produced dizziness and nausea, and I learned to cut the suppository in half. Because suppositories are inconvenient to use, the doctor switched me to oral Cafergot-B, and it was the most helpful treatment to date—as long as I took it at the onset of an attack. I still suffered often, but at least some of my migraines could be aborted. After about 5 to 7 years of use (maybe four pills a week), Cafergot-B was less effective, so the doctor prescribed Fiorinal (with codeine).

Fiorinal worked well in aborting headaches for another 5 to 7 years (maybe three pills per week); again, if triggers were avoided and I took the pill early enough, a migraine could be prevented from developing into a full-blown attack.

About 3 years ago my headaches became nearly constant though generally less severe. Concerned about my increasing use of Fiorinal with codeine, I consulted my doctor and began taking Inderal daily, to see whether it would prevent my migraines. I have found Inderal (240 mg daily, in 40-mg doses) to be an effective preventative migraine medication.

By avoiding triggers, using Inderal, and attending to my muscles (stretching, hot baths, ice packs), I've achieved fairly good control over my migraines. When these methods fail, Fiorinal usually aborts the attack. Although I'm dependent on the medications and have to monitor my food, drink, air, and mood, the results are worth the tradeoff.

My doctor has been as sympathetic and as helpful as I could wish. Whenever I focused his attention on my complaints or on how things had changed, he responded with a new course of action, and he has monitored each new course. Although he doesn't suggest that I pursue every possible avenue relentlessly, I believe he would guide me in any worthwhile approach that I sought. We have discussed all kinds of treatments over the years—headache clinic, therapy, acupuncture—but I haven't wanted to go further or faster than the treatment I've outlined. Chronic states become "normal," and a part of me resists giving migraine any more attention than it has demanded. (Yes, it becomes an entity in one's life, and I resent giving the devil more than its due.)

Migraine clearly has affected my entire life. As a kid, I "failed" in moments of high stress; I was delicate, I was sick, I was weak (I grew ashamed and I learned to hide it). As a teen, alcoholic rites of passage left me heaving on the sidelines (literally). As a young adult, I struggled through parties in pain, smiling but hardly talking or listening, *dying* for a chance to go home.

Even after I learned that alcohol and many foods were the cause of my distress, it took years to say no to friends—no to the toast with champagne, no to the dinner invitation, no to the brie or the soup or the sauce, no to the Mexican restaurant, no to the airline food.

Have family and friends been understanding? Only the few who themselves have had even one migraine, and only the very few who have seen me at my worst. The rest think I'm a fussy eater who can't hold his booze and who is neurotic about eating out. I no longer care whether they are right about me or not. I just say no. I sip mineral water and feast on bread and (undressed) vegetables. I enjoy the company, or I leave quietly. I wish I had learned earlier to take care of myself and to let others take care of themselves.

Bob Weber
New York, New York

Dear Bob:

Your realization that monosodium glutamate (MSG) can be slipped into foods under the cover of such labels as "natural flavoring" or "hydrolyzed vegetable protein" was very astute. According to my research, natural flavorings may include MSG as well as a host of other substances. The MSG in hydrolyzed vegetable protein may have been purified, substantially removed, or remain unaltered. The only way to discover if products using these labels contain MSG is to call the manufacturer.

Dear Betsy:

I am 41 years old, and I have had migraines for 27 of those 41 years. In the beginning, I thought I had sinus headaches. (In the late 60's, I suspect migraines were often misdiagnosed as sinus headaches.)

During my high school years, my migraines were most often associated with my period. Basically, my mother and doctor pooh-poohed them as something I'd have to learn to live with, something akin to a "woman's lot in life."

But once a month quickly became two, three, four, five, six times a month with the headaches lasting anywhere from 24 to 72 hours. I lived with a heating pad on my head and a bloodstream full of aspirin, Extra Strength Excedrin and whatever other over-the-counter medication I thought might help.

Nothing helped.

By the time I was 25, the nausea and the throbbing pain sent me back to my doctor. He diagnosed a possible aneurysm and ordered me to the hospital immediately. Do not pass go, do not collect 200 dollars, do not go home and grab a toothbrush or talk to your small son. Go to the hospital.

The EEG showed nothing, but apparently my reading material spoke volumes. An avid reader, I'd brought along a paperback I was currently reading: *The Electric Kool-Aid Acid Test*. My physician noted the book, raised his eyebrows, and promptly sent in a psychotherapist, Doctor No. 2.

The psychotherapist questioned me about my life but was more interested in the book and eventually dismissed me as a Type A personality. I was "compulsive, overly sensitive, with perfectionist qualities." To soften his diagnosis, he told me "intelligent people get migraines." And then he prescribed Librium.

I didn't take it.

The headaches continued.

I changed doctors.

Doctor No. 3 sent me to Doctor No. 4, an eye, ear, nose and throat man.

Again, nothing was wrong. I was "nervous."

He prescribed Librium.

I didn't take it.

Doctor No. 5 prescribed Fiorinal for the pain. He told me to take up a hobby.

Doctor No. 6 prescribed Fiorinal for the pain and told me to learn to relax.

My husband was killed. Several months afterwards I was very, very sick with a migraine and out of desperation, I went to the emergency room at the hospital. The doctor there said I couldn't "handle stress," and that I had to get myself "together," and learn to "control" myself. Then he prescribed Librium.

Again, I threw the prescription away.

Fifteen years of doctoring, only to be told repeatedly it was all in my head. WAS IT EVER! And in my stomach and in my bowels.

It wasn't just the doctors. My brother-in-law, with his genius IQ, said I didn't exercise enough. He said I needed to jog.

I jogged.

My head pulsated with pain.

No one took me seriously, but rather looked at my headaches as some form of weakness of character.

This past December was the worst month I've ever had. I had a migraine 27 out of 31 days. On January 2, I went to see Doctor No. 8. He listened as I methodically reviewed my history of migraines. He asked dozens of questions and wanted the long version for answers. Finally, he prescribed the beta blocker, Tenormin. He also prescribed the vasoconstrictor, Midrin, and, just in case, Fiorinal for pain.

For 14 days, I have been headache free. *Fourteen days*! I am thrilled, but I am also angry. Angry because virtually every person I know who does not get migraines has patronized me my entire adult life. They believe the nervous, perfectionist, compulsive Type A behavior nonsense. My own husband (I remarried five and one-half years ago) has told me my headaches are due to poor circulation and that they could be remedied if I were to exercise.

The support I needed so desperately from those people closest to me was simply not there. I bought books on headache and underlined all that was pertinent to me, asking my husband to read it. When he didn't read it, I read it to him. He politely listened most of the time. I know he thought, and still thinks, I exaggerate the problem.

I will always resent this attitude. Although it can't make the headaches go away, validation that there is *physical* justification for migraine is important to me. I am not loony.

Migraine triggers for me are stress, sunlight, flickering lights, cigarette smoke, loud noises (particularly *sudden* loud noises), jolts to my head, weather (particularly sudden changes in barometric pressure), and high altitudes. The typical diet triggers aren't really a problem for me unless I seriously overdo them.

The Tenormin is not without its drawbacks. I am more easily fatigued now, but what I have *really* noticed are the DREAMS! They are wild, action packed and, although not nightmares, they are definitely disturbing. I wake up exhausted.

Your book is the most helpful I have ever read on the subject, and believe me, I've read them all. It is comprehensive yet succinct, though not so clipped as to deny the *person* behind the headache.

I think the number one priority for any migraine sufferer should be to find a physician who will treat migraine as the physical malady that it is. I shudder to think what state I might be in had I taken all the Librium prescribed for me by all those "professionals."

This letter is far too long, but it has been *so* therapeutic to "talk" to someone who knows—someone who understands.

If you print this letter, please use only my first name and state.

Again, thank you. Thank you. Thank you.

Betty from Ohio

Dear Betty:

Your letter was very moving. What an ordeal you have been through! Unfortunately, I believe your experience is all too common.

I agree that finding the right physician is most important. Communication with your physician is also important. For example, you might want to ask your doctor if he thinks the side effects you are experiencing with

*Tenormin will diminish with time. Questions about combining your med-
ications would also be appropriate (see the precautions for Midrin in
Appendix I).*

*I admire your courage. With no support, you continued to seek help for
your migraines instead of passively accepting the pain. I know many readers
will identify with your experience and will be encouraged by your strength
to persevere until a proper remedy for their headaches can be found.*

Dear Ms. Wyckoff:

I have the greatest compassion for anyone who has suffered a
migraine at any time in their life, or anyone who is presently suffering from such a curse.

I am 32 years old and have been suffering from migraines for 19
years. I had my first migraine when I was 13 years old. It was a
horrible time. I didn't realize what was going on. At first I would feel
racey. My pulse would rise. I would feel sick and want to vomit but
couldn't. Next, I would lose my vision. Have you ever looked down
a country road in the summer to see the heat rise off the pavement?
Well, when I'd lose my vision that was all that I could see. Being
scared, I would panic, which would intensify the problem. After
about a half hour my vision would return. Then I would suffer the
most massive headache one could imagine.

I was given Fiorinal which took the edge off my headache. I would
withdraw into a dark room or wear sunglasses in the house.

Nobody in my family had ever had a migraine, so they thought I
was faking the pain. My mother would force me to do my daily
routine regardless of my condition. As I grew older my headaches
became progressively worse. The doctor I was seeing used me as a
human test tube, trying to find some medication which worked. By
the time I was 20 years old I was a prescription junkie. Few meds
worked. Most of them just got me over the hump. At one time I was
hospitalized to dry myself out from prescription drugs. The withdrawal symptoms were horrible.

After all the attempts to treat my headaches, I still had migraines.
Finally, I met a heart surgeon who took me on as a patient. As it turned
out, his wife suffered from migraines. She was taking Inderal and it
seemed to work for her. The doctor started me on 40 mg of Inderal
every night at bedtime. Inderal reduced my headaches by about 30
percent. I treat the other 70 percent with strong brewed coffee, two
Wygesic tablets, locking myself in a dark quiet room, and putting my

feet in hot water with a hot pack on the back of my neck. Sometimes I can prevent a full-blown migraine by taking my meds early.

Factors that trigger my migraines are: certain lights, stress, caffeine, sleep, and being frustrated. Sleep and caffeine seem to work both ways.

Thank you for such an informative book.

John L. Hart
Brunswick, Maine

Dear John:

Thank goodness you finally found a doctor who is sympathetic. Have you talked with him about only having a 30 percent improvement in the frequency of your migraines? So many people lose the will to persevere in an attempt to get their migraines under control. For example, it is estimated that over one-quarter of the people who go to a doctor for migraine treatment do not return for a second visit. I do hope that, unlike these people, you will continue to work with your doctor to reduce the frequency of your attacks.

I, too, believe migraine is a curse, but with the right combination of treatments, supervised by a knowledgeable doctor, it is a curse that can be broken.

Dear Betsy:

I have been stranded at work and school, unable to dial a phone for help, and at anyone's mercy too many times not to be extremely grateful for your book.

I am 40 years old and have suffered from mixed headaches for 21 years. My migraines are superimposed upon chronic muscle contraction headaches. A typical headache attack lasts for 3 days and is usually associated with menstruation. I experience pain above my right eye that may be constant or throbbing. Additional symptoms include light and smell sensitivity, vomiting, diarrhea, disorientation, loss of concentration, depression, and chills.

I have identified smoke, car fumes, perfume, glare, and tension as definite headache triggers. I suspect sugar, alcohol, onions, garlic, nitrites, MSG, and food dyes might also be triggers.

I attempt to find relief by resting in a dark room and using a hot water bottle. Acupressure on "hot" spots and foot massage also help. Crying brings relief upon occasion.

I treated my headaches with codeine when they first started, but it spaced me out so much I gave it up. I took so much Excedrin I experienced withdrawal headaches. I am afraid to try Cafergot because the warning label seems worse than the headaches.

My first step will be to look into biofeedback, diet, and exercise as alternatives to drugs. I have contacted the National Headache Foundation for the names of neurologists in my area who also belong to the foundation. I also want to look into the association between depression and muscle contraction headaches.

Thank you for writing this book. You may have saved my sanity.

Mindie Dolson
Oakdale, California

Dear Mindie:

Calling the National Headache Foundation for their physician membership list was an excellent idea. This list will provide you with the names of physicians who are especially interested in headache treatment and prevention. The doctor should be able to give you the name of a local pain clinic offering biofeedback.

Drug warning labels are confusing. We have to remember that the drugs used in headache treatment affect all of us differently. Many people will find a drug benign while others will experience side effects. Migraine sufferers often take a half or a third of a tablet or suppository to see how it affects them before going on to take the prescribed dose.

Migraine triggers can also be confusing. Two triggers may have to be combined in order for a headache to result. This is why amine-containing substances sometimes only trigger a headache when combined with a second trigger (menstruation). When you do not have your period, they may not trigger a migraine.

I am so glad you are taking actions to treat your headaches. Good luck in your search. Mixed headaches are especially difficult to treat and may require a two-pronged attack.

Dear Ms. Wyckoff:

I am a 51 year old, otherwise healthy female, with migraines. I have had migraines since the onset of menstruation at age 11. I'm now through menopause. My headaches have changed "style" through the years. They now appear every 3 to 4 weeks and last for 4 to 5 days. The first 12 hours are very intense. I must close myself in a cool, dark, quiet room and just bear the pain. The rest of the time I try to live with the pain. (I definitely identify with the pictures by migraine sufferers.)

Through the years I've tried all kinds of doctors and have had a variety of tests, including one week at the Mayo Clinic, where I was told that I'm healthy but have migraines, and to keep trying different medicines.

My headaches stopped through each of three pregnancies.

I've tried most prescription medications until I finally gave up and just "accepted" the pain. Because of menopause, I'm now on hormones, which keep my migraines active.

Through a news article I discovered sumatriptan made by Glaxo Inc. I tracked this medication to the Netherlands, where I was able to obtain a package of six tablets. In December, during a full-blown migraine, I took one table of Imigran-100 mg (the Dutch name for sumatriptan). Within one and one-half hours it left completely with no side effects. The headache was gone for 12 hours. This had *never* happened before in 40 years! It is as if I'd never had the headache in the first place. It started again...again I took a tablet. Again it left for at least 12 hours. No side effects. I use approximately six tablets per month. They always work. The effect of this medication is like a miracle. With each pill I've gained 12 to 16 hours of relief, and hope that soon my fellow sufferers will have the same option.

Barbara Neild
Ceresco, Michigan

Dear Barbara:

Glaxo's sumatriptan is an exciting new drug we have all been waiting for with great expectations. It is the first new drug developed in a long time solely for migraine treatment. The injectable form is now available in the United States. Unfortunately, the FDA is expected to take several years to approve the more practical tablet form for use in the United States.

Even with effective medication, we still have to avoid migraine triggers when possible. Because you experience migraines once a month, I wonder if these headaches might be triggered by the days in the month when estrogen therapy is stopped. You may want to talk to your doctor about the noncyclic method in which a low dose of estrogen is taken continuously with no break. Many women find that ERT increases the intensity and frequency of their headaches. A few women, on the other hand, only experience migraines during those days in the month when ERT is stopped. Such is the unpredictability of this disorder.

Once triggers are discovered and removed, we can always take medication to treat the occasional migraine that may occur. Because only a limited amount of abortive medication, such as sumatriptan, can be taken over time, those people who have stopped all known triggers and continue to experience frequent migraines will have to consider preventative treatment.

Appendix I

Migraine Drugs: Dose, Precautions, Side Effects

Only the most common precautions and side effects are presented.
An extremely small percentage of people experience the side effects
listed below. For a complete listing check with your doctor.

ABORTIVE MEDICATIONS

Analgesics
  Aspirin
  Acetaminophen (Tylenol)
  Ibuprofen (Advil, Nuprin, Medipren)
  Tylenol with codeine

Dose:	Follow label for dose. In the case of codeine, take up to 60 mg every 4 hours as needed.[1]
Precautions:	Do not combine analgesics. Do not use ibuprofen with diuretics or if you are taking both a beta blocker and a calcium channel blocker.
Side effects:	Overuse of aspirin and ibuprofen can cause internal bleeding. Stop taking ibuprofen if you experi-

---

1. *Physicians' Desk Reference (1989)*: Oradell, NJ: Medical Economics Co., p. 1244.

ence gastrointestinal bleeding, eye symptoms, rash, water retention, or weight gain.

Comments: To prevent rebound headaches do not exceed 1000 mg of aspirin or Tylenol per day. Codeine should not be taken on a daily basis for any length of time.

Nonsteroidal anti-inflammatory
Anaprox (naproxen sodium)

Dose: 275-825 mg at onset, repeat 275-mg tablet every four hours as needed.[1]

Precautions: Do not use if you are taking Naprosyn, are allergic to aspirin or have kidney disease. Do not use if you are taking both a beta blocker and a calcium channel blocker. Do not combine with diuretics.

Side effects: Nausea, dizziness, itching skin, fluid retention, headaches, drowsiness, abdominal pain, constipation.

Ergotamine
Cafergot
Wigraine
Ergomar, Ergostat

Dose: Oral-2 tablets at onset, may repeat 1 tablet every 30 minutes up to 6 per day and 10 per week.[2]
Rectal-1 suppository at onset, may repeat in 1 hour up to 2 per day and 5 per week.[3]
Sublingual-1 tablet at onset, may repeat 1 tablet every 30 minutes up to 3 per day and 5 per week.[4]

Precautions: Do not take if you have heart disease, high blood pressure, are elderly, have kidney or liver disease,

---

1. Diamond, S. and Millstein, E. (1988): Current concepts of migraine therapy. *Journal of Clinical Pharmacology* 28: 195.
2. Ibid.
3. Ibid.
4. Ibid.

vascular disease, hyperthyroidism, or are taking the antibiotic erythromycin. Do not combine with Midrin or beta blocker.

Side effects: Nausea, diarrhea, pins and needles in hands and feet, elevated blood pressure, leg cramps, abdominal pain, vertigo.

Comments: Daily use can cause rebound headaches. Take with caution during pre-headache aura stage when vessels are constricting. Discontinue use if you experience pins and needles or numbness in hands and feet.

Midrin (isometheptene mucate)

Dose: Take 2 capsules at onset followed by 1 capsule every hour and do not exceed 5 per day or 15 per week.[1]

Precautions: Do not take if you have heart disease, glaucoma, peripheral vascular disease, high blood pressure, severe kidney disease, liver disease, or are taking a MAO inhibitor. Do not combine with ergotamine or beta blockers.

Side effects: Drowsiness, lightheadedness.

Beta-blocker

Inderal (propranolol)

Dose: 10-80 mg per day.[2]

Precautions: Contraindications include heart failure, slowed heart rate, very low blood pressure, breathing difficulties, asthma, severe diabetes, or hypoglycemia. Do not combine with MAO inhibitor. Use with caution if you are combining this drug with a calcium channel blocker. Do not use with Tagamet or ergotamine.

Side effects: Fatigue, nausea, depression, lightheadedness, constipation, insomnia, dizziness, diarrhea, vivid dreams, lethargy, breathlessness.

---

1. Ibid.
2. Peatfield, R. (1986): *Headache.* New York: Springer-Verlag, p. 122.

Caffeine
NoDoz

Dose: 100 to 200 mg per day.
Comment: Do not exceed dose by combining with coffee, tea, or soft drinks.

NAUSEA
Reglan (metoclopramide)

Dose: One 10 mg dose daily.[1]
Precautions: To prevent additive sedative effects do not combine with alcohol, sedatives, hynotics, tranquilizers, or narcotics. Do not use if you are taking a MAO inhibitor.
Side effects: Fatigue, drowsiness, restlessness, anxiety. Dystonic reactions (involuntary movements of limbs and facial grimacing) occur in approximately 1 out of 500 patients treated with 30-40 mg/day.[2]

PROPHYLACTIC MEDICATIONS

Beta blockers
Inderal (propranolol)
Corgard (nadolol)
Blocadren (timolol)

Dose: Inderal: Begin at 80 mg per day and maintain at 160-240 mg per day.[3]
Corgard: Begin at 40 mg once daily and maintain at 40-60 mg once daily.[4]
Blocadren: 10-20 mg twice daily.[5]
Precautions: Contraindications include heart failure, slowed heart rate, asthma, low blood pressure, severe diabetes, hypoglycemia, breathing problems. Do not combine with a MAO inhibitor. Use with caution if

1. Ibid., p. 116.
2. *Physcians' Desk Reference,* op. cit., p. 1704.
3. Diamond and Millstein, op. cit., p. 196.
4. Ibid.
5. Ibid.

you are combining this drug with a calcium channel blocker. Do not use with Tagamet or ergotamine.

Side effects: Dizziness, nausea, depression, lethargy, vivid dreaming, diarrhea or constipation, insomnia, fatigue, breathlessness.

Comment: Discontinue use of drug gradually, not suddenly.

Ergotamine
Bellergal
Bellergal-S

Dose: Bellergal: 1 tablet 4 times a day.[1]
Bellergal-S: 1 tablet 2 times a day.[2]

Precautions: Do not take if you have blood vessel disease, high blood pressure, kidney or liver disease, heart disease, glaucoma, asthma. Do not use with Midrin or beta blocker.

Side effects: Blurred vision, drowsiness, dry mouth, palpitations, urinary retention, flushing, pins and needles in limbs.

Comment: Report numbness or tingling in extremities to doctor.

Antidepressants
Elavil (amitriptyline)
Sinequan (doxepin)

Dose: Elavil: 10-175 mg once daily.[3]
Sinequan: 10-150 mg once daily.[4]

Precautions: Do not use if you have heart disease, epilepsy, glaucoma, or are taking a MAO inhibitor. Do not combine with thioridazine (Mellaril). Check with doctor about using Tagament or drinking alcohol with these drugs.

Side effects: Drowsiness, dry mouth, blurred vision, dizziness, sedation, tingling in fingers, increased dreaming, constipation, urine retention, weight gain, palpitations, lowered blood pressure.

---

1. Ibid.
2. Ibid.
3. Raskin, N.H. (1988): *Headache*. New York: Churchill Livingstone, p. 182.
4. Diamond and Millstein, op. cit., p.196.

Comment: Taper off if taking more than minimum dose.

Sansert (methysergide)

Dose:	2 mg three times a day.[1]
Precautions:	Do not take if you have vascular disease, heart disease, high blood pressure, lung, kidney, or liver disease.
Side effects:	Increased appetite, constipation, insomnia or drowsiness, dizziness, hallucinations, chest and abdominal pain, numbness in limbs, disturbance of balance, fibrosis (scar tissue that forms in heart, lungs, or abdomen), diarrhea, hair loss, weight gain, edema, sweating, nausea.
Comments:	Take test dose of one-half tablet to see if immediate side effects occur. Stop treatment one month out of four to prevent fibrotic side effects. Report pain, coldness, or numbness in limbs, chest pain, leg cramps, and abdominal pain to your doctor.

Calcium channel blockers

Isoptin (verapamil)
Procardia (nifedipine)

Dose:	Isoptin: 80-160 mg three times a day.[2] Procardia: 10-30 mg three times a day.[3]
Precautions:	Take with caution if you have liver or kidney disease. Contraindicated in certain kinds of heart disease. Use with caution if combining with a beta blocker. Do not use with the antihistamine Seldane. Do not combine with calciferol or calcium adipinate.
Side effects:	Dizziness, edema, constipation, nausea, fatigue, headache, lightheadedness.
Comment:	These drugs cause vasodilation and should only be taken when blood vessels are at rest. They should not be taken during the headache phase when the blood vessels are dilated.

---

1. Ibid.
2. Ibid.
3. Ibid.

Appendix II

The Physiology of Migraine: A Recapitulation

In spite of the many theories about migraine, most researchers agree that amines play a role in the development of headache. Some amines, such as serotonin, are made in the body. Other amines are found in the foods we eat. Amines serve many functions, but the one we are most concerned with is their influence on the size of the blood vessels in the brain.

When serotonin is released blood vessels constrict. As serotonin levels fall, the blood vessels dilate, causing pain in the surrounding nerves. What causes serotonin to be released? An increase in estrogen triggers an increase in serotonin. This may be why a birth control pill containing estrogen produces headaches in some women. Conversely, a drop in estrogen levels during menstruation produces a decrease in serotonin, thus triggering vasodilation and headache directly. Stress can also alter serotonin levels. The low blood sugar that results from not eating regularly is another influence on serotonin levels. The amines in the foods we eat cannot be metabolized properly by some people. High levels of these amines trigger a chain reaction that results in vasodilation.

Medications taken once a headache has begun, such as Midrin or egotamine, constrict the already dilated blood vessels, thus eliminating pain. Other abortive medications, such as aspirin or codeine, simply kill our awareness of the pain without reducing the size of the blood vessels.

Some preventative medications, such as the antidepressants, alter the level of serotonin by binding onto serotonin receptors in the brain. By interfering with the entry of calcium into the cells, the calcium channel blockers decrease serotonin release, inhibit vaso-constriction, and dilate cerebral arteries. These medications should be taken only when the cerebral arteries are in a state of rest. If you were to take a calcium channel blocker once a headache is underway, you would be adding dilation to dilation and the pain would be tremendous.

Even without medication you do have some control over your migraine headaches. By eating regularly, eliminating foods containing amines, and avoiding synthetic estrogen and other triggers, the vasodilation associated with migraine can be prevented.

Appendix III

Headache Clinics

Please be aware that the treatment policies of the headache clinics listed below will differ. A clinic directed by a psychiatrist will be more inclined to emphasize biofeedback and other nonmedication modalities. A clinic directed by a neurologist will tend to follow a more traditional medical model. In some clinics, as the eclectic approach becomes more popular, these differences will no longer apply.

UNITED STATES

Arizona
Headache Clinic of the Southwest
1402 North Miller Road
Suite F5
Scottsdale, AZ 85257
(602) 941-5353

California
California Medical Clinic
for Headache
16542 Ventura Boulevard
Encino, CA 91436
(818) 986-4248

Headache Treatment Center of
Orange County
14111 Newport Avenue
Tustin, CA 92680
(714) 832-2505

Neurologic Centre for
Headache and Pain
4150 Regents Park Row
Suite 255
La Jolla, CA 92037
(619) 558-4688

The San Francisco Headache
Clinic
909 Hyde Street
Suite 230
San Francisco, CA 94109
(415) 673-4600

Scripps Clinic and Research Foundation
10666 North Torrey Pines Road
La Jolla, CA 92037
(619) 455-9100

Colorado

Colorado Neurology and
Headache Center
1155 East 18 Avenue
Denver, CO 80218
(303) 839-9900

Headache Clinic of Denver
1355 South Colorado Boulevard
Denver, CO 80222
(303) 759-2220

Connecticut

The New England Center for Headache
40 East Putnam Avenue
Cos Cob, CT 06807
(203) 968-1799

Florida

Headache Management
Center
1925 Mizell Avenue
Suite 100
Winter Park, FL 32792
(407) 628-2905

Headache Management and
Neurology
5500 North Davis Highway
Pensacola, FL 32503
(904) 474-0740

Illinois

Diamond Headache Clinic
5252 North Western Avenue
Chicago, IL 60625
(312) 878-5558

Indiana

Tri-State Headache and Pain Management Associates
801 St. Mary's Drive
Suite 302
Evansville, IN 47715
(812) 473-4394

Kansas

Headache Clinic
Department of Neurology
University of Kansas Medical Center
39th and Rainbow Boulevard
Kansas City, KS 66103
(913) 588-6985

Maryland

Baltimore Headache Institute
11 East Chase Street
Suite 1A
Baltimore, MD 21202
(301) 547-0200

Massachusetts

John R. Graham Headache Centre
Faulkner Hospital
Allendale at Centre Street
Jamaica Plain, MA 02130
(617) 522-6969

Michigan

Department of Neurology
Henry Ford Hospital
2799 West Grand Boulevard
Detroit, MI 48202
(313) 876-2600

Michigan Headache and
Neurological Institute
3120 Professional Drive
Ann Arbor, MI 48104
(313) 973-1155

Minnesota

Headache Institute of Minnesota
2545 Chicago Avenue
Suite G-10
Minneapolis, MN 55404
(612) 870-8066

New York

The Downstate Headache
Center
132 Atlantic Avenue
Brooklyn, NY 11201
(718) 935-9666

Elkind Headache Clinic
20 Archer Avenue
Mt. Vernon, NY 10550
(914) 667-2230

Headache Clinic
Mount Sinai Medical Center
1 Gustave Levy Place
New York, NY 10029
(212) 241-7691

Headache Unit
Montefiore Medical Center
111 East 210 Street
Bronx, NY 10467
(212) 920-4636

Ohio

Headache Department
Cleveland Clinic Foundation
9500 Euclid Avenue
Cleveland, OH 44106
(216) 444-5654

Texas

Dallas Headache Clinic
8226 Douglas Avenue
Suite 325
Douglas Plaza
Dallas, TX 75225
(214) 692-7011

Houston Headache Clinic
1213 Hermann Drive
Houston, TX 77004
(713) 528-1916

CANADA

Ask your doctor to call the Migraine Foundation of Canada in Toronto at (416) 920-4916 for headache clinics in your area. This listing is not available to the public.

UNITED KINGDOM

Admission to the following clinics is dependent upon a referral from your doctor.

England

The City of London	Hull Royal Infirmary
Migraine Clinic	Anlaby Road
22 Charterhouse Square	Hull HU3 2J2
London EC1M 6DX	(0482) 28541
(01) 251-3322	

King's College Hospital	Royal Infirmary
Denmark Hill	Preston
London SE5 9RS	Lancashire PR1 6PS
(01) 274 6222	(0772) 716565

The Princess Margaret Migraine Clinic
Charing Cross Hospital
Fulham Palace Road
London W6 8RF
(01) 471 7833

Scotland
Migraine Clinic
Western General Hospital
Crewe Road
Edinburgh EH4 2XU
(031) 332 2525

AUSTRALIA

Please obtain a referral letter from your doctor before making an appointment.

New South Wales

Department of Neurology	Neurology Clinic
Royal North Shore Hospital	Prince Henry Hospital
Pacific Highway	Anzac Parade
St. Leonards	Little Bay
New South Wales 2065	New South Wales 2036
(2) 438-7111	(2) 661-0111

Queensland
Headache Clinic
Royal Brisbane Hospital
Herston Road
Herston
QLD 4006
(7) 253-8111

South Australia

Headache and Pain Clinic
Queen Elizabeth Hospital
Woodville Road
Woodville
SA 5011
(8) 45-0222

Neurology Clinic
Flinders Medical Centre
South Road
Bedford Park
SA 5042
(8) 275-9911

Appendix IV

Migraine Associations

National Headache Foundation
5252 North Western Avenue
Chicago, IL 60625
In Illinois 1-800-523-8858
Outside Illinois 1-800-843-2256

Migraine Foundation of Canada
390 Brunswick Avenue
Toronto, Ontario M5R 224
Canada
(416)920-4916

The Migraine Trust
45 Great Ormond Street
London WC1N 3HD
England
071-278 2676

Annotated Bibliography

Blau, J.N., ed. (1987): *Migraine: Clinical and Research Aspects*. Baltimore: The Johns Hopkins University Press.

A comprehensive medical textbook on migraine. Each chapter is written by a noted authority in the field. Various theories on the causes of migraine, drug therapy, and nonpharmacological treatments are some of the subjects explored.

Braunwald, E.; Isselbacher, K.J.; Petersdorf, R.G.; Wilson, J.D.; Martin, J.B.; and Fauci, A.S., eds. (1987): *Harrison's Principles of Internal Medicine*. New York: McGraw-Hill.

One of the major texts on internal medicine for physicians. Contains a discussion of disorders that may be accompanied by headache.

Brody, J.E. (1988, October 11): Studies unmask origins of brutal migraines. *The New York Times* C1, C10.

The role of serotonin in the development of migraine is discussed.

Dalessio, D.J., ed. (1987): *Wolff's Headache and Other Head Pain*. New York: Oxford University Press.

A revised and updated edition of a classic textbook on headaches. Two chapters are specifically devoted to migraine.

Diamond, S., ed. (1990): *Migraine Headache Prevention and Management*. New York and Basel: Marcel Dekker.

A comprehensive text for physicians. Chapters are written by well-known headache authorities. Recommended for the reader who wishes to explore in depth the science of migraine treatment and prevention.

Diamond, S. and Millstein E. (1988): Current concepts of migraine therapy. J. Clin. Pharmacol. 28: 193-199.

This article contains a thorough discussion of the abortive and prophylactic drugs currently used to treat migraine.

Diener, H.C. and Wilkinson, M, eds. (1988): Drug-Induced Headache. New York: Springer-Verlag.

Explores how headaches may be caused by the chronic use of some headache medications.

Eisenberg, D. with Wright, T.E. (1985): Encounters with Qi: Exploring Chinese Medicine. New York: Penguin Books.

The autobiography of a Harvard medical student's studies in China. Presents an overview of traditional Chinese medicine in a clear and interesting manner. Available in paperback.

Ferrari, M.D. and Lataste, X., eds. (1989): Migraine and Other Headaches. Carnforth, Lancs. and Park Ridge, N.J.: The Parthenon Publishing Group.

The section on pharmacological treatments is particularly helpful to the migraine sufferer who wishes to investigate the research aspects of drug therapies.

Gallagher, R.M., ed. (1991): Drug Therapy for Headache. New York: Marcel Dekker.

A concise text for physicians. Each chapter is written by one or more specialists in the field. Migraine sufferers would find the chapters on headache triggers, abortive treatment, and prophylactic treatment to be especially relevant.

Glover, V. and Sandler, M. (1990): New developments in the biochemistry of migraine—focus on 5-HT. Headache Quarterly: Current Treatment and Research 1: 174-176.

The association between serotonin (5-HT), selected medications, and migraine is explored.

Hancock, K. (1986): Feverfew: Your Headache May Be Over. New Canaan, Conn.: Keats Publishing.

Written for the general public with many testimonials by people who have been helped by feverfew.

Levine, H.W. (1988-1989): Special report: International congress presents new therapy for migraine sufferers. *National Headache Foundation Newsletter* 67: 1-3.

Glaxo's new drug, GR 43175 (sumatriptan), now undergoing clinical trials, is discussed.

Low, R. (1987): *Migraine: The Breakthrough Study that Explains what Causes it and How it Can Be Completely Prevented through Diet.* New York: Henry Holt.

Explores the role of sugar as a migraine trigger.

Medina, J.L and Diamond, S. (1978): The role of diet in migraine. *Headache* 18: 31-34.

Foods that contain the vasodilator tyramine, and their role as migraine triggers are presented.

Peatfield, R. (1986): *Headache.* New York: Springer-Verlag.

A concise medical textbook written for physicians. The chapters on the clinical aspects of migraine, precipitating causes, the treatment of the acute attack, and preventative measures would be of interest to migraine sufferers.

Physicians' Desk Reference (1993): E.R. Barnhart, publisher. Oradell,N.J.: Medical Economics Co.

The dose, precautions, contraindications, and adverse reactions of all prescription medications available in the United States are discussed in this standard reference.

Raskin, N.H. (1988): *Headache.* New York: Churchill Livingstone.

An excellent medical textbook by a noted headache authority. The sections on precipitating factors and pharmacological treatment are especially pertinent.

Rose, F.C. ed. (1988): *The Management of Headache.* New York: Raven Press.

A research-oriented medical text based on a series of lectures organized by the Migraine Trust and presented to physicians at the Charing Cross Hospital and Westminster Medical School.

Sandweiss, J. (1989): Biofeedback in the treatment of headaches. *National Headache Foundation Newsletter* 70: 1-3.

The author discusses biofeedback and how it can be used to treat tension headaches and migraine.

Steinmetzer, R.V. (1989): Combination drug treatment for headaches. *National Headache Foundation Newsletter* 68: 2-3.

The actions and interactions of drugs commonly used to treat headaches are presented.

Vithoulkas, G. (1979): *Homeopathy: Medicine of the New Man*. New York: Prentice Hall.

A well-written, basic introduction to homeopathy by a world renowned authority and master homeopath. Available in paperback.

Worsley, J.R. (1988): *Acupuncture. Is It for You?* Longmead, Shaftesbury, Dorset: Element Books.

A practical and informative introduction to traditional acupuncture by the founder of the College of Traditional Chinese Acupuncture in the United Kingdom and the Traditional Acupuncture Institute in the United States. Available in paperback.

Glossary

Abortive medication	Medicine that is used to terminate a migraine headache once it has begun.
Acetaminophen	A popular analgesic. Most commonly known by the brand name Tylenol.
Acupuncture	An ancient Chinese method of relieving pain or curing disease by inserting needles into especially designated points in the body.
Amines	Substances found in food or made in the body that serve many functions, including regulating mood and the diameter of the blood vessels.
Analgesics	Drugs used to reduce the awareness of pain.
Androgen	Male sex hormone. The synthetic form of this hormone has been used to treat menstrual migraine.
Antidepressants	Drugs used to alter mood (in depression) and blood vessel diameter (in migraine) because of their ability to control the level of amines in the body.
Antiemetic drugs	Drugs that are used to relieve nausea and vomiting.
Atypical migraine	Gastrointestinal distress, visual abnormalities, or other symptoms associated with migraine may be present unaccompanied by

noticeable head pain. Also called migraine equivalents.

Aura
: Symptoms that precede the headache phase in classic migraine.

Beta blockers
: A class of drugs used to treat people with heart problems. A secondary benefit of these drugs was discovered when heart patients found that their migraine headaches also improved.

Biofeedback
: A method by which people are taught to become aware of their heart rate, blood pressure, muscle tension, and skin temperature in order to consciously control these processes.

Calcium channel blockers
: Drugs that prevent constriction of the blood vessels by interfering with the entry of calcium into the cells.

Chiropractic therapy
: A method of manipulation used to treat headaches resulting from cervical spine disorders.

Classic migraine
: Visual abnormalities, vertigo, tingling, numbness, confusion, nausea, mood changes, or speech disturbances are experienced before the onset of the headache phase.

Common migraine
: No specific symptoms are experienced prior to the headache itself.

Ergotamine
: A fungus that grows on rye that has the ability to constrict dilated blood vessels.

Estrogen
: A female sex hormone. Decreasing levels just before menstruation trigger migraine in some women.

Homeopathic medicine
: A system of health care in which the body's own healing powers are used to overcome disease. Discovered by Samuel Hahnemann in the nineteenth century.

Hypoglycemia
: An abnormally low concentration of sugar in the blood causing such symptoms as headache, sweating, and light-headedness.

Ibuprofen
: An analgesic that has anti-inflammatory properties if taken in a large enough dose.

Brand names include Nuprin, Medipren, and Advil.

Menstrual migraine   Migraine headaches that occur prior to or during menstruation.

Migraine   A headache that is often throbbing in nature and usually confined to one side of the head. Visual disturbances, nausea, and other symptoms may precede or accompany the headache. The pain of the headache phase is caused by dilated blood vessels.

Migraine triggers   Dietary, environmental, chemical, or hormonal substances, as well as emotional factors, that cause a reaction in the body resulting in vasodilation and headache.

Muscle contraction headache   A dull, constant pain that may feel like a tight band around the head. The headache is caused by muscles contracting as a reaction to such emotional factors as stress, frustration, anxiety, or depression. Also referred to as a tension headache.

Neurotransmitter   Chemical released at the junction of two nerve cells that allows or prevents the passing of electrical impulses from one nerve cell to another.

Nonsteroidal anti-inflammatories   These drugs inhibit platelet aggregation which has been linked to the release and destruction of serotonin. They also inhibit certain vasodilators known as prostaglandins.

Octopamine   A vasoactive amine found in citrus that can trigger a migraine in susceptible individuals.

Phenylethylamine   An amine found in chocolate and other foods that can trigger a headache in susceptible people because of its vasoactive properties.

Progesterone   A female sex hormone. Levels of the hormone decrease just before the onset of menstruation.

Prophylactic medication   A medication that is taken daily to prevent migraine headaches from occurring.

Qi	According to traditional Chinese medicine, the energy or life-force flowing through the human body.
Rebound headache	A headache caused by the chronic overuse of such chemical agents as ergotamine, caffeine, and analgesics.
Serotonin	An amine found throughout the human body. Levels of this amine increase prior to a migraine attack and decrease once the headache begins.
Sinus headache	When the sinuses cannot drain properly because of infection or allergy a headache similar to migraine may result.
Status migrainosus	A prolonged migraine attack in which the headache may change in intensity, but never really disappears.
Trager Mentastics	An exercise using dance-like movements to produce a relaxed, meditative state. Used as preventative treatment for the muscle contraction component of the mixed headache syndrome.
Trager psycho-physical integration	A modality used to reduce tension in which the practitioner teaches the patient to use his or her muscles in a less restricted manner.
Tryptophan	An amino acid found in turkey and other foods that is a precursor to the synthesis of serotonin.
Tyramine	An amine found in cheese and many other foods that produces vasodilation and migraine in susceptible individuals.
Vasoconstriction	Describes blood vessels that have decreased in diameter.
Vasodilation	Describes blood vessels that have increased in diameter.
Withdrawal symptoms	Symptoms caused by the abrupt stopping of a drug to which one has become habituated. More of the drug is then taken to relieve the symptoms caused by the cessation.
Yin/Yang	Contrasting forces which together form an interdependent unit.

Index

About the Author

Betsy H. Wyckoff has been a college textbook development editor in medicine, the social sciences, and the humanities for many years. At present, she is a freelance writer. She is an avid art collector and photographer in her spare time.

She majored in premed and English literature as an undergraduate student. More recently, she obtained an M.A. degree in counseling psychology.

Ms. Wyckoff lives in New York City.